How Big Is a Placenta Bowl?

And Other Weird Questions You'll Ask When Planning a Home Birth

Renee Moilanen

CONTENTS

ACKNOWLEDGMENTS

I am so grateful to all of the women and men who spoke with me about their home birth experiences and who graciously shared their advice with others pursuing this path. In particular, I'd like to thank the mothers, doulas, midwives, and childbirth educators from the Yahoo group HAMS (Homebirth and Midwifery Services), which is an invaluable resource for Southern California families seeking natural birth options. And, of course, the biggest thank you goes to Mary Lou O'Brien, CNM, who not only contributed her expertise to this book but also gave me a beautiful, healthy son born in the comfort of our home, which is undoubtedly, the greatest gift of all.

INTRODUCTION

When I decided to have my first child at home, I realized that I was choosing a lonely road. Despite *The Business of Being Born* (the 2008 Ricki Lake documentary that put home birth on the map), high-profile celebrity endorsements, and other efforts to raise its legitimacy, home birth remains a rare event in this country. In 2009, when I had my son, just .72% of births occurred at home, according to the Centers for Disease Control. This percentage was up almost 30% from five years prior, which is a promising sign that more women are choosing home birth, but the numbers are still miniscule.

In other words, if you opt for home birth, you'll have less support and fewer resources than your friends having hospital births. Like I said, it's a lonely road, and you have to be pretty industrious to dig up the information you need.

Don't get me wrong—there are plenty of books out there about home birth. But mostly, I found, these books focus on why you should choose home birth, how it's better for you and your baby, and how the medical establishment has ruined natural childbirth. They often take a motivational, almost spiritual, approach to exalting home birth, and they spend a lot of time focused on the natural childbirth experience. And, quite frankly, they just aren't fun to read.

Believe me, when you're standing in the middle of a store wondering how big a placenta bowl should be, it's pretty amusing, and you realize that home birth has a bigger sense of humor than most books let on.

Plus, once you've already decided on a home birth, you don't need encouragement. What you need is some practical guidance on how to make it happen, the uncensored skinny from actual home birthers, and answers to your most bizarre—and at times, irreverent—questions, like:

- How messy is a home birth?
- How big does a placenta bowl need to be?
- Should I bother getting a tub for a water birth?
- How much does a home birth cost?
- Will my insurance cover it?
- How can I explain to my mother-in-law that I'm not crazy?

This book is a fun and lighthearted attempt to answer those questions. The information comes from mothers who've had home births, including myself, and expert midwives, doulas, and childbirth educators. I also scoured the Web and found other resources to compile everything in one handy guide. There's even a chapter for fathers and partners so they can learn what to expect in a home birth.

This is not a book about pregnancy or parenting, so if you have general questions about those topics, visit your local library and pick up one of the many great books out there. This is a book about midwife-assisted home birth, and I hope you'll let it be your guide to the amazing and transformative experience of having your child in the most natural, beautiful way possible.

Happy birthing!

1

REALITY CHECK

This is not a book about how awesome home birth is, and I'm not going to spend time regurgitating statistics and scientific studies. I don't need to sway you, because you've already read all the books and watched the films (Ina May Gaskin's *Spiritual Midwifery*? Check! *The Business of Being Born*? Check!) I know you can rattle off state-by-state caesarean rates and maternal mortality data from the world's top industrialized nations. After all, we home birthers do our homework.

But because data are so central to our decision to home birth—what conversation with a naysayer doesn't end with the oft-repeated 30% caesarean rate stat?—I wanted to spend a little bit of time putting them in perspective. I'd hate for our community to come across as a bunch of know-it-all home birthers who refuse to acknowledge the risks of an out-of-hospital birth.

Home birth, you'll find, is not a black-and-white issue. Let's not be careless with our use of data. Let's not dismiss hospital-birthers as ignorant masochists. Let's accept what home birth is and what it's not.

Yes, it's true that some studies show better outcomes in home birth compared to a hospital birth; others find just the opposite. Sure, you can pick apart the methods, cry "bad science," and ignore the results. But you'll be doing yourself a disservice. It's simply not accurate to assert that home birth is safer than hospital birth as a blanket rule.

If you read enough studies on both sides of the debate, you'll begin to get the whole picture, which is far more nuanced. Here's the real skinny on home birth:

- Low-risk planned home births have similar outcomes in terms of maternal mortality/morbidity and neonatal mortality/morbidity compared to low-risk hospital births.
- Mothers having planned home births are far less likely to receive interventions, such as epidurals, episiotomies, and caesarean sections, than mothers having hospital births.
- The risk of a potentially injurious or fatal medical emergency occurring during a planned home birth is extremely low.
- If such an emergency occurs, your outcomes are likely to be *worse* at home than in a hospital.

This isn't rocket science, and I'm not trying to freak you out, but it's good to understand the facts so we—members of the home birth community—don't become cavalier about this nontraditional choice. If you have a low-risk pregnancy and a qualified midwife, you'll most likely have a wonderful home birth. If, on the other hand, you encounter an emergency that requires immediate medical intervention, you'll be in worse shape.

Again, the risks of a problem are small. Postpartum hemorrhage, which is a significant factor in maternal mortality, occurs in about 4% of vaginal deliveries (and incidentally, having an episiotomy is a major risk factor). Cord prolapse—when the umbilical cord slips into the cervix and gets compressed by the baby—is a serious and life-threatening condition but occurs in only .1% to .6% of all births. Many times, it is preceded by an intervention you'd never find in home birth, such as artificial rupture of your membranes.

These risks should not dissuade you from a natural birth at home. But they're a good reason to find a qualified midwife, identify back-up obstetricians, and have an emergency plan in place.

Also, by keeping the home birth experience in perspective, you can address concerns from your friends and family without sounding like you drank the crazy Kool-Aid. Despite all your stats, people won't believe: "Home birth is safer than hospital birth." But they'll accept: "For a low-risk pregnancy like mine, home birth is just as safe as a hospital birth and a more comfortable experience for Mom and Baby."

So be pragmatic. Be realistic. And don't get caught up in proving yourself. At the end of the day, the best validation of your decision is the beautiful, healthy birth of your new baby. When that happens, the statistics won't matter at all.

And now, it's prep time!

2

AM I CRAZY?

Congratulations, you've decided to have a home birth! Bask for a few days in the warm glow of female empowerment, then take a good look in the mirror and ask yourself: Am I crazy? Because if you're being honest, the answer is, yeah, a little bit.

You've just chosen a path taken by fewer than one in 100 women. It's a great path, but you need to know what you're getting into. Before you get swept away by the euphoric high of reclaiming a womanhood lost to Western medicine, it's worth asking yourself some tough questions. Some of them are practical—like, can you afford a home birth?—and others are more philosophical, like do you have the right temperament for this experience?

A good midwife will ask you many of the questions that follow or at least try to suss out the answers in conversation. But consider them now before you get too far down the road.

Do you have a low-risk pregnancy?

Home births have great outcomes in part because they start with low-risk pregnancies. If you have a high-risk pregnancy, your best bet is in a hospital. Don't feel bad about this! We're fortunate in our society to have highly skilled obstetricians and fantastic medical facilities that make high-risk pregnancies possible. What constitutes a high risk? Home birth is not a good option if you have high blood pressure, preeclampsia, diabetes, a history of preterm births, or if you're at risk for a preterm birth now, according to the American Pregnancy Association.

Other conditions may also rule you out, including a breech presentation. Some midwives will not attempt a home birth if you've had a previous caesarean section, otherwise known as vaginal birth after caesarean, or VBAC. And if you're having an active herpes outbreak when you go into labor, you'll need to go to a hospital.

I'm pregnant with twins. Should I rule out home birth?

Not necessarily. Some midwives will perform a home birth for multiples. But others won't. Aside from personal preference, your midwife may be prohibited by state law from attempting a home birth for twins, so you'll need to check your state's regulations.

With a single birth, the baby engages in the pelvis at the start of labor, which means there's little risk of a breech presentation or the umbilical cord slipping into a dangerous position. The same holds true during delivery of the first twin. But the second twin can't engage in the pelvis until the first one's out, so there's a greater chance something could go wrong. I'm not saying it will. But the risks are higher in a twin birth.

You'll need to have a long conversation with your midwife and spend some time assessing your tolerance for risk. If you decide to forge ahead, find a midwife with experience delivering twins at home and have a good back-up obstetrician in case things don't work out the way you'd planned.

Do you have quick access to a hospital?

Almost always, home births go as planned. But if something goes wrong, it's important to know that you're a short drive to the local emergency room or that paramedics can be at your house within minutes. Generally, you should be no more than 30 minutes from a hospital by car (which will be much shorter by ambulance). I was fortunate to live no more than 10 minutes away from two great hospitals. Knowing that I could get help quickly if necessary gave me a lot of reassurance and made my decision to birth at home much easier.

Are you physically able to handle the demands of natural childbirth?

The short answer is, of course you are! Women's bodies were made to give birth. But labor can be grueling and exhausting, and you should be able to handle the physical exertion. You don't need to be a marathoner, but you should be in reasonably good shape. If you have any concerns or specific medical conditions, discuss them with your midwife in advance.

Are you mentally prepared for birthing at home?

It's hard to know if you're prepared for something you've never done before. But there are a few personality traits that seem to bode well for home-birth success.

The home birth moms I've spoken to over the last few years are the most confident women I've ever met. And that's not a coincidence. You simply must have faith in your body to birth a baby naturally. When I was pregnant, people would bombard me with questions: "What if something goes wrong? How will you deal with the pain? What if you need an epidural?" And despite the fact that I'd never before had a baby, I would answer: "I just know it's going to be okay." And I was certain of it. I just *knew* that my body could do it, my baby could do it, and my midwife could do it. Confidence is critical.

Home birthers also are very good at knowing when to exert control and when to let things happen organically. If we're being honest, all of us home birthers are control freaks to some extent. I couldn't stand the thought of nurses or doctors telling me what was best for my own body, and I loathed the idea of ceding control to a hospital staff. But at the same time, so much of a home birth is letting go. You need to let your body do what it's going to do. You need to let your baby take the lead. You need to trust in nature. If you struggle with that balance, home birth may be a challenge for you.

And lastly, home birth may not be the best choice for hypochondriacs. The reasons seem pretty obvious, but if you need more explanation, read on.

I keep worrying that something will go wrong. Is this normal?

I've got news for you—every expectant mother worries that something will go wrong, including (and maybe especially) women planning hospital births. The difference is that if in the very rare event that something goes terribly awry, we home birthers don't have immediate access to the high-tech lifesaving measures available in a hospital. That's nothing to take lightly, so in a sense, yes, it's normal to consider the unexpected.

But rest assured, midwives are prepared for emergencies. Contrary to public perception, they don't show up at your house with a bucket of hot water and some towels. They carry all sorts of lifesaving medical supplies, and in most cases, they'd perform the same exact procedures you'd receive in a hospital under similar circumstances.

That said, if you feel as though you are *preoccupied* by thoughts of something going wrong, maybe home birth isn't for you. You need to have confidence in your body, your care team, and your ability to birth a baby without medical assistance. A little bit of worry is normal; anxiety is not.

Is your home an appropriate space for labor?

Assuming you don't live in a cardboard box, your home is probably fine. But do a quick assessment to make any changes well before your labor starts. Make sure you have comfortable places to relax—couches, chairs, beds—not just for you, but also for your midwife and her assistant, who may be there a few hours while you're laboring. And if parking is a challenge in your neighborhood, think about how you'll secure a spot for your midwife on the day you go into labor so she's not circling the block while your baby is crowning.

If your house gets uncomfortably cold, get a space heater. If your house gets too hot, buy a few fans. You'll need running water and telephone service with 911 capabilities (sounds like a joke but a lot of

Internet phone providers don't automatically equip you with emergency access). If you're planning a water birth, make sure the tub is big enough to hold you and your massive belly *and* give your midwife plenty of room to maneuver. Otherwise, you'll need to rent a birthing tub.

Your home should be clean. Don't worry about scrubbing behind the refrigerator with a toothbrush (although you may find yourself doing that when those nesting hormones kick in), but if you're the kind of person who leaves food rotting on the kitchen counter or hoards broken bicycle parts in your living room, you may want to straighten up.

Lastly, you may want to think about your neighbors, especially if you live in an apartment, condominium complex, or dense townhome development. One fellow home birther suddenly found the cops at her door because the neighbors heard screams and thought she was being beaten by her husband. Feel out the situation. If you have a close relationship with your neighbors, you might want to mention it. But don't feel as though you need to flier the apartment complex or put it on the agenda of your next homeowners association meeting.

Is your partner supportive?

I couldn't have imagined going through labor at home without a supportive partner. My husband was a rock star. He kept me hydrated, fed, and focused for the 27 hours I was in labor. When I was at my wit's end and telling him I couldn't do it anymore, he reminded me that I could. His certainty gave me renewed strength; if he'd expressed any doubts, I probably would've crumbled.

Your husband, boyfriend, or partner is key to your success. You're going to face a lot of scrutiny over your decision to birth at home, and you'll have your own concerns. You need someone to stand up for the decision you've made as a couple and to help you put those worries aside. If your partner is unsupportive of a home birth, you may want to consider a compromise, such as having your baby in a birth center or pursuing a natural birth in a hospital with the aid of a doula. But I would strongly advise against home birth if you don't have a willing partner.

Can you afford home birth?

There are three main costs in a midwife-assisted home birth:

1. the midwife fee, which includes pre- and postnatal care and the birth itself, usually including her assistant,
2. birth supplies, and
3. laboratory tests.

If you decide to have a water birth, you may also incur costs for renting or buying supplies, and the services of a doula would be extra.

The midwife fee varies greatly by location, but the range is around $2,500 to $4,500. Expect to pay more in cities (as high as $7,500 in places like New York City), less in rural areas. Midwives with more experience often charge higher rates. Some lay midwives—particularly those who assist home births as a religious calling—may charge nothing at all. In general, plan to pay around $4,000 for the midwife fee. Insurance may cover some or all of this fee (see Chapter 9 for more information on insurance), but you should be able to swallow the whole cost just in case it doesn't.

Although the midwife will bring medical-grade supplies, you'll be responsible for buying the birth kit, which contains cord clamps, underpads, iodine, and other products needed for birth (more on the birth kit later). You can buy these online for $25-$35. You'll also need to provide additional materials, like plastic sheets, garbage bags, and towels. Most of this stuff you can get around the house, but you may need a trip to the dollar store. Figure about $40 total for birth supplies.

Lastly, if you choose to have prenatal testing, there are laboratory fees. Most expectant moms will get, at minimum, a blood test for gestational diabetes and a swab for Group B streptococcus. If you want an ultrasound or amniocentesis, you'll be referred to a medical facility, where you'll be subject to their prices. Lab tests are almost always covered by insurance (make sure the lab is in-network) so real costs are hard to assess. But without insurance, ultrasounds may range from $500 to $800, and blood work could be around $100. Again, insurance coverage for lab work is rarely an issue.

So the grand total for a home birth is somewhere around $5,500. You may not get your insurance company to pay for much of it, so make sure you can swing the cost. If that's a challenge, see if your midwife will work with you on price or offer a payment plan. Some midwives might even barter if you have enticing services to offer her.

Given the lack of insurance coverage, your out-of-pocket costs for a home birth likely will be a lot more than what you'd pay for a hospital birth (even though the actual cost of home birth is about one-third of a hospital birth), which is why the resurgence in home birth has primarily occurred among middle- and upper-class women. Yes, home birth is expensive. But it's totally worth it.

3

HOME BIRTH ISN'T FOR HIPPIES

When I was pregnant, I dreaded answering questions about my childbirth plans. Inevitably, an acquaintance would ask: "What hospital are you using?" And I'd have to stammer out an answer. "Well, I'm not actually going to a hospital, I'm having a home birth, and well, you know, I'm not crazy, and I'm not a weird hippie or anything like that, I just, you know, wanted a natural experience ... " And as I rambled on, this poor unsuspecting sap would nod her head, smiling awkwardly, and inch slowly away from the crazy lady with the tinfoil hat.

Home birth, although on the rise, is a rarity in this country. And if you opt for home birth, you have to be prepared for people to think you're nuts. Get over it now. Don't get indignant about the snide comments you might receive or bemoan the sad state of our medicalized society. Don't condescend to women who've had their babies in hospitals or — horror of horrors — opted for an epidural. You may feel empowered and enlightened by your decision, but 99% of American women think you're a loon, and once you've accepted that, you can move on.

Unless you're surrounded by like-minded friends who think home birth is just peachy keen, you'll need to figure out a way to deal with the questions and comments that come up. Over the course of nine months, I honed my skills answering questions about home birth and defending my decision. Your responses likely will vary depending on who's asking.

In some circumstances (like when a random pedicurist asked which hospital I was going to), it's just easier to lie. Give them the name of a local hospital and change the subject. No need to touch off a socio-political discussion with a stranger especially with all those hot-headed pregnancy hormones racing through your body.

Many times, people are just curious. When people hear "home birth," they may picture hippies, the ultra-religious, and hillbilly rubes, certainly not the well-adjusted, professional woman before them. The reality is that most home birthers today are white, college-educated, and nonsmoking women in their 30s and 40s making an informed decision to reject hospital birth.

People may need some time to reconcile their preconceived notions with reality. They want to learn more about your decision to birth at home, and it's a great opportunity to advance the cause, answering questions openly and honestly.

Other times, people may act hostile toward you, as if threatened by home birth. This was a reaction I hadn't anticipated. But some women, in particular, seem to feel as though having a natural nonhospital birth somehow diminishes their own birth experience (it doesn't, and you need to reassure them), and they get downright bitchy about it.

And then there are the toughest critics — your relatives. These folks need the most convincing that you've not gone off the deep end. You can't brush off their concerns or lie to them. You need to answer their questions, assuage their concerns, and sometimes, just let them vent.

I've compiled a list of the most common offenders and advice on how to deal with them drawn from my own experience and those of other home birthers. You'll need to assess your own comfort level with answering questions about a rather personal, and in some ways, intimate experience, but these profiles provide a starting point.

The Pedicurist

This is the random stranger who unknowingly stumbles onto the home birth land mine. It'll start with an innocent question from your pedicurist/grocery clerk/barista such as, "So when are you due?" You'll answer, hoping you can steer clear of any more discussion. But they forge on: "What hospital are you using?" At this point, you have two options.

If you have time to spare, you can tell them you're having a home birth, but believe me, you'll be there answering questions for a while. If you don't want to deal with it (and I rarely wanted to deal with it), just lie. Tell them you're going to XYZ Hospital. They'll make some comment about how their sister-in-law went there and loved its great new birthing center, yadda, yadda, yadda, and you can nod your head in agreement, grab your latte, and sneak out before the questions get tougher.

The Overly Excited Interrogator

This person is genuinely awed when you mention home birth. She'd never dream of doing it herself, but she's open-minded enough to see how other people can do it, and she'll be excited to tell you all about this documentary she saw, you know, the one with Ricki Lake … (yes, we've all seen it). She'll have tons of questions for you, but she asks them in a nonthreatening way, and it's a pleasure to answer them. Most people, in fact, fall into this category. You'll leave this conversation feeling renewed and encouraged by your decision to birth at home.

The Stephen King of Birth Stories

When this person finds out you're having a home birth, she immediately launches into the most horrific, gore-filled, tragic birth stories you've ever heard. Babies getting lodged in birth canals, gruesome perineal tears, massive hemorrhaging — you name it, and she's known someone who lived through it. She's a virtual anthology of vaginal delivery gone wrong. Her goal is to make you feel stupid and irresponsible for choosing home birth. I used to try to rebut the horror stories. If a person tells you about a forceps delivery that resulted in a gushing wound to the baby's head, you really want to rail about the misuse of forceps and the reckless haste to use high-tech interventions in hospital births. But it'll get you nowhere.

So instead, when someone started telling me a horrific birth story, I'd say, "Wow, and that happened in a home birth?" At which point the person would look flustered and say, "Well, no, it happened in a hospital." To which you can smugly respond, "Hmm, sounds like a hospital is just as dangerous."

Hostile Mom aka "The Topper"

If you spent 30 hours in labor, hostile mom spent 31 hours. If your baby weighed 8 pounds at birth, hostile mom's baby weighed 8.5 pounds. If you had a slight perineal tear, she ripped open like a zipper. The point is, whatever birth experience you had, hers was much worse, which is why she never could have had a home birth, and frankly, the only reason you had one is because your birth was a piece of cake.

This woman clearly has issues about her own birth experience, and it results in a hostile "topper" mentality designed to diminish your accomplishment. When hostile mom hears that you plugged through two days of labor with no painkillers, she feels bad about getting the epidural. So she'll say something like, "Well, my baby was so much bigger than your baby, of course you were able to go without drugs. Try delivering an 8-pound baby without an epidural."

Look, this isn't a competition. And it's unfortunate that natural childbirth has developed a "badge of honor" stigma as if we home birthers are deliberately trying to show up the moms who got epidurals. Who cares? I never argue with hostile mom. Instead, I say, "The babies all come out one way or another—as long as they're healthy." And that usually shuts her up.

Your Family

Your relatives are a tougher sell. They have almost as much invested in that little fetus as you do, and they want to make sure everything's going to be okay. Since they're of an older generation (and because they probably haven't seen *The Business of Being Born*), they'll think your decision is outlandish and irresponsible.

They'll pose a ton of what-ifs. What if the baby stops breathing? What if you can't get to a hospital in time? What if you start hemorrhaging? They'll try horror stories (see "The Stephen King of Birth Stories"). And they'll do everything they can do to change your mind, holding onto any shred of hope that even at the 11th hour, you might come to your senses and go to a hospital.

You can't blow off your relatives, so you'll need to answer their what-ifs and address their concerns. One home birther took her mom to a natural childbirth store for a screening of a documentary about home birth. Her mother was able to learn about home birth in a non-threatening forum and to meet other couples choosing home birth. This savvy home birther also sent a copy of the film home to her dad so he could better understand her decision.

But you also need to be very clear about your intentions every step of the way. Don't give your family false hope that you'll change your mind. When my in-laws found out that I'd met the back-up ob/gyn, they were ecstatic. A real live doctor! "So he can deliver the baby? You can go to him during labor?" they asked, gushing with relief. I had to explain to them, very patiently, that I would only see the doctor if something went wrong. Our intent was to have our baby at home with the midwife. End of story.

Needless to say, many conversations ended in stony silence.

It's hard, but sometimes, you just need to be firm. At one point, after some seriously passive-aggressive naysaying, I finally had to say, "This is our decision, our choice, and you don't have a say in it." By the way, family pressure is another reason why it's so critical to have a supportive husband—then they can't divide and conquer.

So your family, by far, is your toughest audience. Be patient with them. They love you. They love your unborn baby. They're sick with worry. Reassure them, and when you're holding that baby in your arms after a problem-free home birth, make sure they're the first people you call.

4

THE MOST IMPORTANT DECISION YOU'LL MAKE

The single most important decision you will make — after opting for a home birth — is choosing your midwife. To this day, I revere my midwife as some sort of demi-goddess who enabled me to bring my son into the world in the most natural and beautiful way possible. It is a gift for which I will be eternally grateful.

Finding the right midwife is a very personal decision. You may want someone with a strong medical background and experience working in a hospital setting, someone who can—and will—perform more advanced interventions if necessary, such as suturing, an episiotomy, and setting up an IV drip. Or you may want someone who favors aromatherapy, herbs, and more nontraditional approaches. Educational credentials might matter to you. Maybe they don't. That's your call.

But above all, your midwife must be a good fit for you and your family. Many times, that just comes down to a feeling you get about her. Is she easy to talk to? Does she inspire confidence in her skills? Do you have any reservations at all about using her? And don't feel bad if you don't love the midwife that everyone's gushing about. Sometimes, personalities just don't sync up, and that's okay. Keep looking for the midwife who makes you feel at ease.

That said, you also need to temper your expectations. A midwife is not a doula, and she's not your birth coach. She's not going to sit and hold your hand for the 20 hours you're in labor. She's not going to bring you tea and massage your back. She's not there for emotional support (although that will be a byproduct of her presence). She's there to deliver your baby. And you want her completely focused on that task. If you need support during childbirth, hire a doula or make sure you have a strong network of friends or family willing to help out. But let your midwife concentrate on what she does best — delivering healthy babies to healthy moms.

When looking for a midwife, you first need to decide what type of midwife is right for you. Then, you need to know where to find them. Lastly, you need to narrow down the list and find the right person to lead you on this incredible journey.

Types of Midwives

Your head will spin with the alphabet soup of midwife designations out there. Do you want a CNM or a CM? Is a CPM the way to go? What the heck is an LM? Adding to the confusion is the fact that each designation has its own credentialing, education, and training requirements, and they're all viewed differently in the eyes of the state, which may license some types of midwives but not others. The type of midwife you choose also matters to your insurance company, which may cover charges from some designations but not others.

All midwives, regardless of designation, adhere to a similar philosophy that pregnancy and birth are normal life events. They'll provide you with prenatal and postnatal care and hands-on assistance during labor and delivery, and they'll minimize high-tech interventions. So really, it comes down to formal training and education, and, of course, your own read on a potential midwife.

For basics, there are two main categories of midwives: certified nurse-midwives and direct-entry midwives. Certified nurse-midwives, or

CNMs, have the highest degree of training and formal education (bachelor's degree and master's degree in midwifery required), and they can practice legally everywhere. Direct-entry midwives, or DEMs, may or may not have formal education.

Twenty-seven states permit direct-entry midwives to practice with a license. Ten states explicitly prohibit DEMs, and the rest of the states are a gray area in which these midwives are legal but unlicensed. I've included a table at the end of the book that describes some of the state-by-state regulations governing midwives.

For more details on the types of midwives, read on.

Certified Nurse-Midwives

A Certified Nurse-Midwife (CNM) is a registered nurse with a graduate degree in midwifery. They must pass a national certification examination to receive the designation. There are about 12,000 CNMs in the country, and most of them work in hospital settings; just 3% offer home births. On the plus side, this hospital experience means that many CNMs have witnessed complications in childbirth, giving them first-hand knowledge of how to deal with problems in a home birth should they arise. CNMs are the only midwives who are licensed to practice and prescribe medication in all 50 states and the District of Columbia. Almost all private insurance companies will cover services provided by a CNM. They're certified by the American College of Nurse-Midwives.

Direct-Entry Midwives

Direct-entry midwives are regulated on a state-by-state basis, which means each state has different rules about how they can operate, whether or not they can administer or prescribe medication, and whether insurance companies are mandated to cover their services. The Midwives Alliance of North America maintains a great matrix showing which states regulate direct-entry midwives and under what conditions. You can find it at www.mana.org.

Most states that license direct-entry midwives permit them to carry drugs commonly used for childbirth, including oxygen, Pitocin (a potentially lifesaving drug if you're hemorrhaging), Rho(D) immune globulin, and local anesthetics. Some states, however, allow only oxygen or nothing at all. Midwives in these states may carry the drugs regardless of the law, but your midwife will have better legal protection—and so will you—if she has the authority to do so. When in doubt, ask your midwife what drugs she carries with her. Only one state, New York, allows direct-entry midwives to prescribe medications outside of those required for childbirth.

I used a CNM, which was handy, especially when I developed a breast infection a few weeks after birth, and my midwife was able to quickly call in a prescription for antibiotics. But many direct-entry midwives have good relationships with other health care providers who can provide non-emergency medication if necessary. You'll need to check with your state's licensing board to find out the specific restrictions that apply to direct-entry midwives in your area.

Direct-entry midwives are less likely to be covered by private insurance. Using a direct-entry midwife licensed by your state is your best bet for getting coverage, but even then, it's no guarantee.

Certified Midwife (CM)

A Certified Midwife (CM) is not a registered nurse but has a bachelor's degree and usually a background in another health-related field or at least completion of select science courses. CMs must receive a master's degree from an accredited midwifery education program and pass the same national certification examination as CNMs. Because it's a fairly new designation, there are only about 70 CMs in the country. Most practice in hospitals and health centers.

CMs are currently legally able to practice in five states: Delaware, Missouri, New York, New Jersey, and Rhode Island, which means they're afforded the same legal protections and authority as CNMs. They're able to prescribe medication in New York. Many private insurance companies will cover services provided by a CM; coverage is required in the five states in which they're authorized. They're certified by the American College of Nurse-Midwives.

Certified Professional Midwife (CPM)

A Certified Professional Midwife is a knowledgeable, skilled and independent midwifery practitioner who's been certified by the North American Registry of Midwives (NARM). There are about 1,800 practicing CPMs. Many of these midwives do not have formal midwifery education. There are two pathways to becoming a CPM: graduation from a midwifery school or an apprenticeship under a qualified midwife who attests to the prospective CPM's skills. According to NARM's most recent survey, about 45% of CPMs came through the apprentice model.

Regardless of their background, all CPMs must pass a written examination to receive the designation. CPM is the only credential that requires knowledge about and experience in home births. States that regulate direct-entry midwives are increasingly using CPM as the de facto credential. Insurance companies are less likely to cover a CPM, but some will. Most CPMs can administer drugs commonly used during childbirth, including Pitocin for hemorrhaging, but the laws vary by state.

Lay Midwife

Lay midwives are uncertified or unlicensed midwives who were educated through informal routes such as self-study or an apprenticeship rather than through a formal program. Lay midwives may be just as skilled as their counterparts but for whatever reason chose not to become certified or licensed. If you use a lay midwife, you're not likely to get the charges covered by your insurance, and they may be limited in the services they can provide.

You might also hear the term "licensed midwife" or LM. This just means the midwife is licensed to practice in your state. You'll need to probe further to find out her credential. If your state licenses midwives, it's a good idea to use one who is licensed. It affords you and her more legal protection and could help in securing insurance reimbursements.

The bottom line is, if you're confused about a midwife's background and the specific credential she holds, ask her about it. She'll be happy to explain her training and qualifications.

Where Do I Find a Midwife?

The Midwives Alliance of North America (MANA), through its sister Web site, www.mothersnaturally.org, has a search function to locate midwives in your area. But the list that comes back is crude. You can't tell which midwives practice home birth; many of them may only work in birth centers or hospitals. Plus, in order to get listed, midwives must be members of MANA. It's worth noting that when I did the search, my midwife's name did not come up, nor did the names of some of the other more popular home-birth midwives in Los Angeles.

Like everything else in life, referrals are the best way to find a midwife. But with less than 1% of births taking place at home, the chances of you knowing another home birther are, well, 1 in 100. This doesn't bode well for referrals.

So start by reaching out to natural childbirth advocates. HypnoBirthing instructors, Bradley Method practitioners, prenatal yoga teachers, doulas—these folks are well tapped into the home birth network, and they'll be happy to toss a few names at you. Seek out a breastfeeding support group or a store that caters to alternative-minded parenting (think baby wraps and co-sleepers). Gather more names. Find an online group dedicated to home birth and midwifery.

Also, although it seems counterintuitive, ask an obstetrician or gynecologist. When I asked my (entirely unsupportive) ob/gyn for a home birth referral, she reluctantly gave me the name of the midwife I ended up using. At the very least, you may learn which midwives don't have great reputations in the medical community because of poor care or high transfer rates.

After a while, you'll start to hear the same names over and over again. Once you have an initial short list, it's time to make some calls.

Is She the Right Fit?

The only way to find out if you like a midwife is to meet her and ask a few questions. Almost all midwives will give you this opportunity. In fact, I'd have reservations about using a midwife who refuses to meet with potential clients in advance. For that kind of service, you could've stuck with your ob/gyn.

That said, there are some ground rules for interviewing midwives. First, you don't need to interview every midwife in a 30-mile radius. Maybe just two or three tops. (There are probably only two or three in your area anyway.)

Second, make sure your husband or partner attends the meeting, because it's important that he or she also feels comfortable with the midwife. In my experience, husbands are far less interested in the interview than the mother, but it's good to have them there anyway.

Third, be respectful and appreciative of the midwife's time. Midwives are extremely busy. Between delivering babies at all hours of the night and seeing women for prenatal appointments, midwives also provide follow-up care for newborns and their moms. Plus, they have their own families and social lives. Yes, it's important that you get the answers you need, but the midwife has real paying clients that require her attention, so don't monopolize four hours out of her day and then hire someone else. Spend an hour—tops—on the interview.

Lastly, remember that the midwife is interviewing you as much as you're interviewing her. She'll be on the lookout for signs that you might be difficult to satisfy, hard to work with, or litigious, and she also wants to know that you both are on the same page in terms of philosophy and expectations. Even though you'll be paying her, the midwife is more partner than employee. So be sure to get off on the right foot.

During the interview, you can chat with the midwife informally or bring some prepared questions. I've compiled some questions from various resources, including the Web, other midwives, home birth moms, and my own wished-I-would-have-asked-that list. I've also provided some suggested answers, or, at least, some considerations.

But you don't need to treat the interview like an interrogation. Remember, you're trying to get a general sense of who the midwife is and how she operates. Do you feel comfortable talking to her? Does she make you feel at ease? Do you have confidence in her? It's important to feel a connection to your midwife. You'll be spending a lot of time together—and some pretty intimate moments—so make sure she's a good fit.

That said, there are some very basic things you should expect from your midwife, a sort of checklist that can start the discussion. For me, these would be deal breakers if the midwife balked.

Your midwife should:

- Be certified as a CNM, CM, or CPM with formal training and experience in home births.
- Be licensed by the state and in good standing with the licensing board. Your state can tell you whether the midwife has ever had any restrictions put on her license.
- Have first-hand experience as the primary midwife in home births (more on experience later).
- Provide prenatal care throughout the pregnancy and postnatal care for at least six weeks after your baby is born.
- Have a back-up ob/gyn with whom she consults if concerns arise and to whose care you can transfer if necessary.
- Have a back-up midwife to care for you in case your primary midwife is on vacation, sick, or has another mom in labor when you're ready to give birth.
- Visit your home 3 to 4 weeks before your due date to check out the facilities and supplies and to note any concerns.
- Agree that you generally should be able to do what you want in labor—move around, try different positions, eat, drink, rest.
- Bring an assistant with her to the birth.
- Conduct a physical examination of the baby after birth.
- Accompany you to the hospital if you need to transfer.
- Never be judgmental about your choices. If you want to have an amniocentesis, vaccinate your baby, or have your son

circumcised, your midwife should not belittle your decisions or put undue pressure on you to change your mind. If you start to feel uncomfortable, it may be time to switch midwives.

Once you've checked off this list, you can move on to some other questions.

How many births have you attended as the primary caregiver?

Your midwife should have hundreds of births under her belt. That's right, I said *hundreds*. The reason is that in home birth, complications are very rare. A midwife might see a true emergency once every 150 births or so, and you want to know she can handle it. Plain and simple, experience matters in home birth, and sheer numbers are the way to get there. If you think large quantities are tough to achieve, keep in mind that a lot of midwives worked in hospitals or birth centers where they saw huge volumes of births, so 500 deliveries isn't a tough number to come by. And even a moderately busy midwife doing 50 births a year can rack up 200 or 300 births in a relatively short amount of time.

When you ask this question, make sure the midwife gives you the number of births at which she was the *primary* midwife, not the number of births she's attended or served as an apprentice. If a youngish looking midwife is telling you she's done 1,500 births, question her on that number.

Also, if it's relevant, you'll need to know how many twins your midwife has delivered. Again, experience counts, and you don't want to be her first attempt at a twin birth.

How many births are you attending now? Do you have a maximum, and how do you manage to avoid too many commitments?

A moderately busy home birth midwife does 3-6 births a month. But that's at least one birth a week on top of her prenatal and postnatal visits and round-the-clock schedule. For most midwives, the sweet spot seems to be around three or four births a month or about 40 a year. Most midwives will stop taking clients with similar due dates when they feel overcommitted. Your midwife's caseload is important.

It's one thing for your midwife to miss a birth because she's sick or on vacation. But if she has a habit of missing births because she's overcommitted, you don't want to be the client left stranded.

How do you handle emergencies? Under what circumstances would you transfer? Have you ever had to resuscitate a baby?

Basically, you want to hear the horror stories. You want to understand what she considers an emergency and what her response would be, and you want to know that she can handle a variety of complications should they arise. I was a fairly neurotic pregnant mom, and even though I supported home birth, I was very pragmatic about the potential risks. I wanted a midwife who wouldn't take chances, someone who wouldn't hesitate to intervene or even transfer my care to a hospital if she had any concerns about my health or the baby's health.

In the hundreds of home births she'd done, my midwife had seen two emergency transfers to hospitals, and both resulted in good outcomes for mom and baby. Information like this didn't tell me anything about my own likelihood of facing an emergency. But I read a few things into it.

For one, my midwife was probably good about screening out high-risk situations, even risks that occurred later in pregnancy, such as a breech presentation or preeclampsia. This was important, because it showed she had a conservative approach. Second, my midwife was likely able to handle a lot of complications on her own, such as postnatal bleeding. This is important, too, because you don't want your midwife cracking under pressure. Less experienced midwives have higher transfer rates, so again, look for a midwife with a lot of successful births.

In the end, you just want to get a sense of the midwife's approach and experience. It won't tell you a lot about your own risk, but it will give you comfort in knowing that she's dealt with emergencies in the past and would be ready for them in the future.

How many women whom you have attended have had to go to the hospital?

Home birth transfer rates are funny things. If you look at national studies, you'll see percentages anywhere from 7% to 40%. That's because transfer rates can include a whole lot of things—true hair-raising emergencies, less urgent hey-it's-better-if-we-just-go-to-the-hospital incidents, and moms who just poop out and want an epidural. Some published transfer rates also include moms who transfer out of midwife care before labor even begins. So if your midwife gives you a transfer rate, the number itself may not tell you much.

Instead, ask general questions. How many moms go to the hospital because they can't take it anymore? If it's a fairly high percentage, maybe the midwife doesn't do a great job preparing moms for the rigors of childbirth, or maybe she doesn't offer enough comfort in labor, such as IV fluids. How many moms transfer because of emergency situations? If it's a high number, it may indicate that your midwife doesn't have the right experience to deal with complications.

Still, you need to keep the midwife's answers in perspective. She's not likely to have hard and fast data to share with you, only estimates. But even anecdotal responses can help you form an impression of her abilities and your likelihood of success.

If I require a transfer to the hospital, will you accompany me?

If you're going to the hospital, your midwife should go with you. End of story. Whether or not she stays with you for the long haul is another question.

In emergency situations, where your life or the baby's life is in jeopardy, your midwife should stay through the end to make sure everyone is safe and healthy.

But if you're going to the hospital because you're tired and want pain relief, some midwives might leave once they know you're settled and comfortable. Remember that most home-birth midwives have no hospital privileges, so they cannot intervene on your behalf or even make recommendations to the hospital staff. In the hospital, your midwife effectively becomes a doula or a friend. You could be in labor for another few hours, and maybe her time is better spent with other clients.

Still, many midwives will stay with their client until the baby is born and breastfeeding, regardless of the circumstances. If that's important to you, make sure you ask this question.

What interventions would you use or have you used? How often?

Home birth midwives want to give you an intervention-free birth. They're not going to rush to do an episiotomy. They're not going to strap you to a fetal heart monitor. They won't automatically start an IV line. It is their goal to avoid such interventions. That said, in some circumstances, midwives may need—or want—to intervene, and you should understand your midwife's perspective on such interventions from the outset.

For example, some midwives may suggest IV fluids if you're getting dehydrated or may break your amniotic sac to augment labor. Most will want to monitor the baby's heartbeat during labor, usually with a fetal Doppler. If you're not comfortable with some or all of these interventions, you need to let the midwife know up front.

For example, I knew a midwife who routinely used a Doppler during labor to monitor the baby's heart rate. One potential client refused. The midwife, feeling as though she wouldn't adequately be able to gauge the baby's health, declined to take on the client. No hard feelings.

I will say, however, that you should think twice before digging in your heels against all interventions in all circumstances. Midwives are experts at what they do. They want to avoid interventions. They want you to have a natural birth. If you tie their hands, they can't do what they do best, which is delivering healthy babies. It's simply not realistic to expect the midwife to sit idly by while you're laboring. If you are against intervention at all costs, you should consider an unassisted home birth.

Tell me about the prenatal care you provide. How long do these visits last? What do they typically involve?

When I was interviewing midwives, I was fixated on the labor and delivery part of home birth. I asked all the questions you'll see here—what if there's an emergency? What sort of interventions do you use? What's your transfer rate? But looking back, I realize that the birth itself, although very important, was the smallest part of my experience with the midwife. Far more significant were the countless hours she spent with me during my prenatal visits.

Your midwife should provide comprehensive prenatal care on a regular schedule throughout your pregnancy with increasing frequency towards your last trimester.

During a typical prenatal visit, your midwife should:

- check your weight
- take your blood pressure
- test your urine
- evaluate the baby's position and fundal height (a measurement of your uterus designed to assess fetal growth)
- listen to the baby's heartbeat with a fetoscope or Doppler
- ask you questions about your nutrition, activity, and general physical condition
- advise you on what you should be doing at this point in your pregnancy
- answer your questions

Your midwife also should be able to conduct herself or refer you to someone who can perform common prenatal tests including:

- blood screens for sexually transmitted diseases and genetic disorders
- glucose tolerance test between the 24th and 28th week of pregnancy to check for gestational diabetes
- culture for Group B streptococcus (GBS), which can be harmful to the baby

- ultrasound
- amniocentesis

My midwife blocked off an hour for each of her prenatal visits, and I was usually there about 45 minutes. When's the last time your doctor gave you 45 minutes of his undivided attention?

Do you carry malpractice insurance?

Some states require midwives to carry malpractice insurance. Others do not. In states where malpractice insurance or professional liability is not required, most direct-entry midwives do not carry it. If your midwife doesn't carry malpractice insurance, she may ask you to sign a waiver in which you acknowledge the risks of home birth and the fact that she doesn't have liability coverage.

Can I contact some of your clients?

If you didn't find your midwife through a referral, you might want to talk to some of her past clients. The midwife might feel uncomfortable handing over their information, but she'll probably pass along your name and number. Then it's up to the past clients to contact you. But believe me, we home birthers are thrilled to talk about our experiences—we'll call.

Undoubtedly, the midwife is only going to refer you to clients who had good experiences. That's okay. At least you'll be able to talk to the moms to learn more about the midwife's approach and to hear about their experiences (plus, it's a great way to meet other home birthers!)

Other Considerations

In addition to the questions above, there are some other things you should consider when hiring a midwife.

Check to see if your midwife is covered by your insurance. Chances are, she won't be, but it's worth asking. If your midwife is in network, you could save big bucks. Also, ask your midwife if she'll take care of billing the insurance company. Very few home birth midwives will get involved with insurance companies, but it's a huge help if they will.

Consider how far away your midwife works. Given the scarcity of home birth midwives, you may not find someone right down the street. But it's not a good idea to use a midwife who's really far away. For one, you're going to need to see her pretty often for prenatal visits, once a week toward the end of pregnancy. If she's far away, it's going to get tiresome. Second, once you go into labor, you want her to be able to get to you quickly because you never know how fast you'll advance.

There's no hard and fast rule on how far is too far. But generally, your midwife should be within 30 miles and roughly able to get to you in 30 minutes. Even with traffic, it should take less than an hour. That may limit your options in rural areas or car-clogged places like Los Angeles and New York, but it's better to be safe than sorry.

Getting Down to Business

After you've chosen your midwife, you need to formalize the arrangement. Your midwife likely will require a monetary deposit, which reserves your spot. Once she gets too many due dates in a particular month, your midwife may stop taking clients, so it's important she knows you're committed. Usually this deposit gets credited toward the total fee at the end of the pregnancy.

Your midwife should have you sign a contract; if she doesn't, you should suggest it. The contract should include her price and exactly what this price covers. For example, does it include the fee for her assistant? The newborn blood screen? A birthing tub? Also, the contract should spell out the payment plan, if any. And it will probably include some language that you're responsible for paying the bill whether or not insurance covers it.

The contract may also include some unique terms and conditions. For example, one midwife makes her clients agree to at least attempt breastfeeding. Another requires first-time home birthers to hire a doula and restrict the number of friends and family attending the birth.

Such provisions aren't likely to be a hard sell to most home birthers, but there may be other terms and conditions that give you pause so give the contract a good read.

Also, don't be surprised if your midwife makes you sign an acknowledgement that she does not carry liability insurance and a waiver of claims against her if something goes wrong. The provision sounds harsh, but many home birth midwives do not have malpractice coverage, and the waiver of claims is common practice.

Now that you've got your midwife, and everything's squared away, it's time to relax, enjoy the next nine months, and prepare for the birth of your baby.

5

NATURAL CHILDBIRTH WON'T KILL YOU

About a year after I gave birth to my son, I went to a friend's baby shower. All the ladies sat around in pretty party dresses, balancing trays of canapés on our laps, oohing and aahing over adorable baby clothes. The conversation turned to childbirth, and soon, the women were sharing their atrocious birth stories.

One woman remarked, "I had a natural birth."

"Really?" said another. "You didn't have an epidural?"

"Oh no, I had an epidural," the first woman said. "But not a c-section." (Note: Because of our country's abysmal caesarean rate, many women now think "natural" birth means a vaginal delivery. It doesn't, but more on that later.) Then she added, "I don't know *anyone* who doesn't have an epidural." The other ladies nodded in agreement.

At this point, my pregnant friend said, "Renee didn't have one." Now I was outed as the freak who spurns Western medicine.

The women looked at me with a mix of horror and surprise.

"Well," sniffed one of the ladies, "I was in labor for 14 hours. Fourteen hours! I needed the epidural." (This woman was clearly a "topper" mom). She turned to me: "How long were you in labor?"

I replied. "Twenty-seven hours."

The women were abuzz. They couldn't fathom labor without painkillers. They really couldn't see—it wasn't even in their mindset—how anyone could stand it. Surely, I must have had an easy labor (I didn't) or I was some sort of pain-tolerant she-beast (I'm not).

These days, using pain medication during labor is the *default* option. And when you choose to reject it, as you will in home birth, there will be women at every turn trying to convince you that it's not possible.

Here's the thing. It is possible. And it happens all the time.

Society makes an incredible hoopla over the pain of labor. It's become a terrible cliché ("It was worse than labor!") and spawned hundreds of bad analogies (i.e. if you want to know what childbirth feels like, stretch your bottom lip up over your head). So if you feel anxious about it, that's expected. You'll be motivated to prepare yourself.

Personally, when I was pregnant, I didn't dwell on the pain of labor because I figured there wasn't anything I could do about it. Maybe it was my own good fortune that I'd never before had a baby so I didn't know any better. But to this day, when people ask how I survived a long labor without drugs, I shrug and say, "It is what it is."

You want a home birth? You want a drug-free experience? You want all natural? You have to take it all—every contraction, every pulse of pressure, every ache—and know that it's your body and your baby working in perfect harmony.

Of course, there are strategies you can use to minimize your discomfort, which I'll describe later, and you should avail yourself of them. But even before you sign up for HypnoBirthing classes or rush off to prenatal yoga, put childbirth in perspective and give yourself a little pep talk.

You've committed to a natural birth.

Contrary to an increasingly popular misconception, a natural birth does not mean delivering a baby through your vagina (although that's part of it). A natural birth means you're not strapped to a fetal heart monitor with an IV in your arm and a catheter in your spine. It means you won't use any artificial pain killers. And yes, it means you'll deliver vaginally. The lack of unnecessary interventions makes for a healthier baby and mom, but you might not appreciate this upside when you're in the throes of labor. Embrace it now. You're going to sacrifice a little bit of comfort for the greater good. Welcome to motherhood.

Everyone has a different experience.

Don't let your nosy co-worker terrorize you with her labor stories—it has nothing to do with your labor. Everyone experiences childbirth differently. Some people have a higher pain tolerance than others. Some people's bodies simply respond better to stress. And who knows what another person's "pain" feels like? I spoke to one woman who said labor felt as though her insides were being ripped out, and another who said she felt no pain at all, just a heavy pressure. Maybe they were experiencing the same sensation—there's no way to know. So don't fixate on what others tell you about the experience, because yours will be unique.

It's not bad pain.

Driving an ice pick into your eye is excruciatingly painful. And worse, you'll lose an eye. Labor, on the other hand, feels exactly the way it's supposed to feel, and everything goes back to normal when you're through. In other words, the discomfort is temporary, normal, and healthy. You can't compare it to painful disorders or traumatic injuries, and don't let anyone else do that either. When you're in labor, remind yourself: this is exactly what my body is meant to do.

When you don't think you can go on anymore, congratulations!

Almost every woman reaches the point where she thinks, "I can't do this anymore." For me, it was around hour 24. When you're having intense contractions and you watch the sun go down, rise, and go down again, it can get pretty demoralizing. I remember soaking in the tub and saying to my husband, "I don't think I can do this anymore." I must've looked awful because he consented to calling the midwife. I told her: "I need you to come over and check me. And if you tell me I'm 5 centimeters, I'm going to the hospital and getting an epidural." This was my rock bottom.

Little did I know but this was a great sign! When my midwife arrived a few minutes later, I was a solid 9 centimeters. The end was in sight, and it renewed my spirit. In fact, many childbirth methods, including The Bradley Method, identify this phase—sometimes called "self-doubt"—as the time when women need the most encouragement, because they're almost there. So when you think you can't do it anymore, it probably means you're near the end, and that should be reason enough to forge on.

You won't remember it.

It's an old cliché but very true: After some time, you probably won't remember the pain. A 2008 study out of Sweden found that five years after childbirth about half of women reported their childbirth as far less painful than they did two months after the birth. The more satisfied a woman was with her birth, the more likely she was to forget the pain (as an interesting aside, women who had epidurals were far more likely to report intense pain than those who didn't have one, possibly because they were remembering "peak pain"). So whatever you're feeling in the moment, or even a day later or weeks later, don't worry—you'll soon forget.

It is what it is.

This is my old standby, and it works. Childbirth is what it is. No sense worrying about it. Trust me, you *will* find a way to deal with the discomfort, and it will come to you effortlessly. Just keep yourself open to it.

When in doubt, use external motivation.

One home birth mom made a bet with a friend that she'd make it through natural birth unscathed. The friend, incredulous that anyone could withstand labor without drugs, said, "I'll bet you end up with an epidural." The mom took her up on it and bet a dollar she'd make it without an epidural. "After I had the birth, I went and collected my dollar from her," the mom said.

Getting Prepared

All that said, it's a good idea to prepare for natural childbirth. You wouldn't show up for the New York Marathon without having trained for a while, and you certainly wouldn't forget your running shoes.

You can start by learning techniques to improve your mindset and to encourage relaxation during childbirth. Being relaxed is a huge help in labor. When you're stressed and anxious, your body tightens and causes more discomfort. But when you let go of that tension, your body eases into submission.

There are tons of childbirth education modalities out there, and you'll need to find the one that works best for you. Some require formal classes; others you can read about and practice on your own. Personally, I liked having a structured class, because I was able to ask questions and hear from other pregnant couples, but it's up to you.

Also, you might want to consider some tools to help you stay more comfortable during labor, like physioballs, aromatherapy, and baths. You won't know what will work for you until the contractions hit, but it's good to know your options.

Childbirth Preparation Options

Most hospitals offer childbirth preparation classes that discuss the birth process and skills to help with labor. But these classes likely will not spend much time on the strategies you'll need for a true natural birth because the audience is primarily women having hospital births, about 60% of whom will have an epidural. So my recommendation is to seek out childbirth preparation modalities that assume you'll have a drug-free birth and that provide you with real coping strategies.

Natural childbirth education classes have a few things in common. Almost uniformly, they:

- describe the birth process (although each method may use different terminology),
- emphasize relaxation in labor based on the premise that tension increases pain,
- incorporate breathing techniques as a way of staying relaxed,
- encourage different positions during labor and delivery (not just lying on your back), and
- teach birth partners how to be active supporters throughout labor.

What makes each method unique is the extent to which it emphasizes some of these points more than others.

Below, I've described the four most popular methods acutely focused on natural birth. I'm sure there are instructors who have their own spin on these methods and even totally different ideas about birth preparation. But these are the major methods you should be able to find in every city.

The Bradley Method

The tagline for The Bradley Method is "husband-coached natural childbirth." This method really emphasizes the role of the birth coach (typically a husband, but it could be anyone). You and your husband will learn how to care for yourself during pregnancy, what to expect when you go into labor, and how to cope with discomfort. Husbands will learn how to support and be an advocate for you, and they'll learn relaxation techniques and effective labor and birth positions. The goal is to educate and motivate coaches and make them a valuable part of the birth experience.

The classes are 12 weeks long with 3 to 6 couples per class and include a 130-page workbook, labor rehearsals, and role playing. Most couples start around the fifth month of pregnancy. If it seems like a long commitment, remember that these classes also include information about breastfeeding and parenting, so you may be able to skip some of the other classes you were going to sign up for. The organization claims that nearly 90% of Bradley Method moms having vaginal births do so without pain medication.

Key concepts:
the six needs of the laboring woman: darkness and solitude, quiet, physical comfort, physical relaxation, controlled breathing, appearance of sleep and closed eyes; emotional sign posts to guide you through labor's phases

Kook factor:
You'll get instruction on "emergency childbirth"—what to do if you give birth in a car or before the midwife gets there.

For more information or to find an instructor:
www.bradleybirth.com

HypnoBirthing

HypnoBirthing is based on self-hypnosis, promoting the idea that you can relax deeply enough to feel little (or even no) pain during labor. HypnoBirthing starts from the premise that fear creates anxiety in moms-to-be, which in turn, leads to the sensation of pain during labor. For this reason, this method advocates letting go of fear and replaces the entire lexicon of childbirth with new words. Contractions become "surges." Pain becomes "tightening" or "pressure." Water breaking becomes "membranes releasing."

There are four main techniques: breathing, relaxation, visualization, and deepening. There are five class sessions with 3 to 6 couples per class, and it comes with a HypnoBirthing book and a CD with guided meditations. You'll be expected to practice the breathing and relaxation techniques on your own.

I used HypnoBirthing for my birth, and while I wasn't skilled enough to avoid pain, I was extremely relaxed during labor. In fact, my midwife doubted my progress because I sounded too composed every time I called her. But to be fair, the guided meditations and New Age music were a bit much for my left-brained husband, who thought the whole thing was flaky.

Key concepts:
breathing, relaxation, visualization, and deepening; letting go of fear

Kook factor:
You'll be asked to visualize your contracting uterus as a ball of unfurling blue ribbons and to "breathe your baby down" instead of pushing.

For more information or to find an instructor:
www.hypnobirthing.com

Lamaze

Don't dismiss Lamaze because it reminds you of your mother's generation. Lamaze is the original "breathe-breathe-breathe" childbirth method, but it's come a long way since the 1950s and now encompasses a much broader, home birth friendly philosophy of avoiding medical interventions, changing positions during labor, and not birthing from your back.

And yes, there's the breathing. Lamaze teaches you to breathe differently at various stages of labor. You'll begin and end each contraction with a cleansing breath—a big sigh—and switch to shorter inhales and exhales during more intense contractions, sucking in with a "hee" and exhaling with a "hoo." This pattern creates the "hee-hee-hoo" mantra that's so often referenced in pop culture.

Classes are 12 weeks long and may have up to 12 couples in a class. You can often find Lamaze classes or some variation of them in hospitals. Many midwives also are certified in Lamaze.

Key concepts:
relaxed breathing, using different positions to find comfort during labor, not birthing from your back

Kook factor:
You'll become a natural birth cliché with your "hee-hee-hoo" breathing.

For more information or to find an instructor:
www.lamaze.org

Prenatal Yoga

Prenatal yoga isn't really a childbirth preparation class because it rarely involves formal instruction. Since there's no "classroom" component, you won't learn the details of the birth process or specific strategies during each phase of labor, but prenatal yoga classes are a great way to practice relaxation, breathing, and getting in tune with your body and baby. The classes also feature customized stretches and poses designed to aid in childbirth.

While the other methods will help you get mentally ready for childbirth, yoga also prepares you physically by strengthening muscles needed in labor and by releasing tension that could manifest itself as pain during labor.

Key concepts:
deep relaxation breathing (pranayama), mindfulness, stretches and poses to reduce discomfort and to ease into better birthing positions

Kook factor:
You'll practice poses with names like "butterfly," "warrior II," "tree," and "fish."

For more information or to find an instructor:
Locate a yoga studio or instructor near you through the Yoga Alliance, www.yogaalliance.org. Not all studios offer prenatal yoga, so be sure to ask in advance.

Comfort Aids

The classes will prepare you for childbirth, but when you're in labor, you may need all the help you can get. Consider having some tools on hand to provide a more comfortable position, release tension, or just take your mind off things. I've listed a few of the most common tools here. Doubtless, there are others.

Birth Ball (aka exercise ball)

You've seen these giant inflatable balls at the gym or in Pilates class. Some women find them helpful during labor because they provide support but also yield under your weight. The ball also allows you to rock easily from side to side. Two of the most common positions are sitting upright on the ball with your upper body draped over a chair or bed, or kneeling beside the ball and stretching your chest and arms over the top. But there are no rules, so find whatever position works for you. You can pick up an exercise ball for under $20 at your local sporting goods store or discount retailer.

Birthing Stool

These low stools with the seat cut away enable you to get into an assisted squat. Squatting is probably the best position for pushing out a baby. Some midwives report more perineal tearing in women who sit on the birthing stool for a prolonged period of time, so it should be used with caution. Your midwife might have a birthing stool for you to use. Otherwise, you can buy or rent one. Honestly, I've never known anyone to use a birthing stool. A more common choice is to have your partner support you in a squat with his arms looped around your chest. But birthing stools are an option if you feel they might be helpful.

Baths and Showers

Water can be a godsend during labor. Soaking in a tub or taking a shower can relieve pressure, release tension, and re-energize you. This comfort is why many home birthers choose to have a water birth, actually delivering their baby in a large tub. But even if you don't want a water birth, you can use baths and showers to ease your discomfort. I was in and out of the tub multiple times during my labor and even took a shower at one point (mostly because I was feeling grungy after so many hours). I was surprised by how much it helped. Some words of advice: have someone assist you getting in and out of the tub. The last thing you want to do is slip and fall. And make sure someone is always within shouting distance while you're soaking.

Aromatherapy

Surrounding yourself with pleasant aromas can be a welcome distraction, and some scents may even speed the natural birth process. Buy the scents as essential oils, which you can find at most health food stores. Put a few drops of the oil on a cotton ball and set it by your bed, or wherever you're laboring. The nice part about having it on a cotton ball (as opposed to putting it on your skin) is that you can easily remove the aroma if you get sick of it. According to aromatherapy experts, jasmine and lavender produce calming effects, geranium rose enhances circulation and breathing, and myrrh speeds labor and opens the cervix.

Massage

Massage relieves tension and just plain feels good. Coax your birth partner into rubbing your head, shoulders, feet, wherever it helps.

Water Birth

Many home birth mothers choose to have water births, and why not? Soaking in the water is a natural form of pain relief. The buoyancy lessens your body weight so you can move freely, and the water alleviates stress-related hormones. Plus, as a home birther, you have the option, so take full advantage of it.

Admittedly, I didn't have a water birth, mostly because I dreaded the thought of one more logistical challenge. And to be fair, some moms experience unexpected hiccups when setting up or filling their tubs, so you'll need to be prepared for additional work. But if I had to do it over again, I'd go with a water birth because I found the water very helpful as a form of pain relief. Most of the mothers I spoke to had water births, and they all raved about it.

When considering a water birth, first assess whether your home bathtub is adequate. You should have enough room to spread your legs, and your midwife must be able to maneuver in and around the tub. This usually rules out many of the bath-shower combos because the shower doors or faucets get in the way.

Also, you need to make sure the water will cover your abdomen completely once you're in it. If the tub is too small, you won't get sufficient water coverage. In general, the freestanding jacuzzi tubs meet these criteria, but if you have doubts, ask your midwife. She might suggest you rent a birthing tub.

Birthing tubs, or birth pools, are designed for water birth. They're spacious enough to hold you and your partner. They're compact enough to fill quickly. And they're sturdy enough for you to brace against during a particularly tough contraction.

These tubs can be as simple or as fancy as you want. You can get a tub with a built-in seat and thermal linings. Or, if you want to save money, just go to the toy store and buy a big inflatable wading pool. The bottom line is, as long as you can sit comfortably with ample water coverage and your midwife can move around, it should be fine. Word of warning: If you go the cheaper route and buy a kiddie wading pool, remember to buy it in spring or summer. You won't have any luck finding one at your local retailer in the dead of winter.

You can rent a birthing tub and its associated supplies from your midwife or doula, or you can buy one. Sometimes the cost runs about the same, but you probably won't have much use for a birthing tub once the baby's out, which makes rental an attractive option.

I've outlined the water birth supplies in Chapter 6 and how to set up the tub in Chapter 7. But here are a few tips on water birth:

- Practice setting up the tub ahead of time. Your husband or partner probably will be the one getting it ready on labor day, so make sure he has tested the parts in advance and knows how to inflate and fill it. Some rental companies will come to your house and set up the tub for you. If your husband isn't especially handy, you might want to take them up on it.

- Consider your hot water tank. One home birth mom ran out of hot water when the water level was only ankle deep. They frantically started boiling pots of water, but the temperature never got above lukewarm, and her midwife was concerned about delivering the baby in tepid water. Eventually, they went ahead with it and everything worked out, but it's good to have a Plan B. Keep in mind, you might need about 130 gallons of water to fill your birth tub. So if you can't make it through a 15-minute shower (about 37 gallons) without using up all the hot water, you'll need to get those pots boiling.

- Test your water pressure. Like the hot water tank, weak water pressure could foil your plans for a water birth. It can take anywhere from 40 minutes to 3 hours to fill the larger birthing tubs depending on your water pressure. If you have a slow flow, plan ahead and start filling the tub early.

Do I Need a Doula?

Doulas help you prepare for and carry out your birth plans, and they'll stick with you throughout labor. They provide emotional support and physical comfort, and they'll take pressure off your husband or birth partner.

In a hospital birth, doulas play a critical role of improving communication between you and the medical staff and of advocating on your behalf to make sure the medical staff doesn't push unnecessary medical interventions. The doula's role changes in a home birth, where you won't face pressure to have interventions, and in fact, won't even have the option. But they still provide a lot of value.

A doula will help you get comfortable. She knows little tricks to get your labor to progress. She can give your husband a break if he needs to get some fresh air. Basically, they're paid to focus solely on you—and that's a pretty good deal.

Midwives also like having doulas around. Remember, the midwife is focused on making sure you and the baby are healthy. She doesn't have time—nor is it her job—to hold your hand, wipe the sweat from your brow, and make you a cup of tea. In that sense, a doula also takes pressure off your midwife, freeing her up to concentrate on your health and safety.

You should choose a doula in much the same way you'd choose anyone on your care team. Find someone with whom you feel comfortable, someone who makes you feel at ease, someone who will instill a sense of confidence in you and your abilities. Your partner also needs to be comfortable with your doula.

You should make sure your doula is certified through a recognized program, such as DONA International, the International Childbirth Education Association, or the Childbirth and Postpartum Professional Association (CAPPA). Certification demonstrates that your doula has formal training and knowledge of the birth process.

To find a doula, you can start with the organizations noted above. Most of them have searchable databases of their members. Or, you can reach out to other moms, childbirth educators, and breastfeeding support groups for referrals.

Once you've identified a few potential doulas, interview them. Feel out their perspective on birth. Get a sense of how they would interact with your husband or partner. Make sure you'd feel comfortable with them participating in this very personal and intimate experience.

Unlike midwives, in which the sheer number of births is important, the quantity of births attended by a doula is far less critical than how you feel about her. So don't rule out someone with only a few births under her belt. She may be just the right fit for you.

A doula's services are not included in your midwife's fee, and they vary by location (higher prices in cities, lower prices in more rural or suburban areas). A doula could run you anywhere from $300 to $1,200, and the average is around $500.

And if you'd rather go it alone, that's okay, too. In childbirth, it's all about your comfort level. Letting go of expectations is an important part of the natural birth experience.

6

I NEED A *WHAT*?

There was a moment—as I tossed old towels, shower liners, and birth supplies into a cardboard box—when I thought, "What the heck am I doing?" I was going to have a baby. *In my house.* And I'll admit, it was just plain weird to prepare my home for an event that rarely occurred outside the sanitized, highly contained walls of a state-of-the-art medical facility.

It was even weirder for my friends, who'd marvel at my growing collection of medical pads, cord clamps, garbage bags, and lube. The presence of my birth kit—a tangible representation of what I was about to do—made it all very real. And pretty funny.

"A placenta bowl?" one friend asked, reviewing my checklist. "You need a *placenta bowl*?"

Believe me, you'll have many strange moments when prepping for home birth. But embrace it now, because preparation is the key to home birth. You don't want to be sitting there with a newborn baby in your arms and realize that no one packed the cord clamps.

In addition to gathering supplies, you'll need to make some decisions about the birth, such as, do you want your other children present during the birth? What happens if you need to transfer to a hospital? What are your preferences? And you'll need to think about decisions made after the birth, such as, do you want to circumcise your boy? Depending on the answers, you may need to do some prep work in advance.

What follows is a guide on how to prepare for the big day, from gathering birth supplies and lining up specialists to making sure you have food in the fridge. And I've also answered the irreverent and bizarre questions that only home birthers ask themselves.

The Birth Kit

Let's face it, as it stands now, your living room is no place for a baby to be born. That's why you need a birth kit. Before rushing out to buy 70 yards of plastic sheets, talk to your midwife. She'll give you specific instructions on what she wants in your birth kit. Some midwives bring things like gloves and baby weighing scales; others don't.

Several online stores sell birth kits with more of the hard-to-find, medical-grade supplies. Cascade HealthCare Products and In His Hands Birth Supply are two big names in home birth kits. These kits include:

- bulb syringe
- lubricating jelly
- cord clamps/tape
- gloves
- iodine/hibiclens scrub (antiseptic)
- sanitary brief
- various sizes of underpads (chux pads)
- plastic-backed sheets
- sanitary pads
- perineal irrigation bottle
- gauze

- alcohol prep pads
- flexible straws
- infant tape measure
- basic infant cotton cap

Some midwives create customized birth kits they'll want you to purchase, either through them or one of the companies mentioned above.

But that's just the beginning. You'll also need to get some items on your own. Many of these things you can find around the house. Start now collecting old towels, sheets, and wash cloths. For other items, make a trip to the dollar store or discount retailer. When it comes to home birth supplies, don't spend a lot of money because you'll be throwing most of it away.

- garbage bags
- freezer bags
- scissors
- old towels, wash cloths, and blankets
- two sets of sheets (you'll throw out one set after the birth)
- bowl for the placenta
- cookie sheet
- 2-3 plastic sheets or shower curtains (disposable plastic-sided tablecloths also work)
- more lubricant and/or olive oil
- more sanitary napkins
- newborn diapers
- baby receiving blankets
- flashlight
- mirror
- map to the nearest emergency room
- contact information for the nearest hospital, back-up obstetrician, and pediatrician
- birth plan (if you have one)

Some midwives might also want you to get some herbal remedies, like tea tree oil, which can help reduce perineal infection after birth. So again, check with your midwife.

Once you have all these items collected, throw them in a large cardboard box or laundry basket and store them in one easily accessible location. Store your comfort aids, such as birth balls and essential oils, in the same spot. You should have everything collected and stored at least six weeks before your due date.

If you're planning on renting or buying a birthing tub, you'll need to get some additional supplies.

- birthing tub
- tub liner (buy some extras if you intend to try out the tub before labor)
- air pump
- water thermometer
- small fishing net for light debris removal
- hose with universal adapter to attach to the faucet

Usually, you can rent or buy all of these supplies from one store, and for a proper birthing tub, it'll probably run you around $250 for a three-week rental. You can buy everything for about the same cost. If you go with a plastic kiddie pool, you're looking at about $30.

As you get closer to your due date, you'll need to make sure your kitchen is stocked. You should have coffee and food on hand for your midwife and assistant in case they're at your house awhile as you labor.

But you'll need to eat, too. You're probably not going to scarf down a hamburger between contractions, but you should eat and drink as much as possible.

Opt for soft, easy-to-eat foods, since your body will be doing enough work:

- Coconut water

- Gatorade or other sports drinks
- Yogurt
- Cottage cheese
- Honey
- Soft fruits

Also, make sure you have ready access to a car with gas in the tank in case you need to go to the hospital. Ideally, the car will have room for you, your partner, your midwife, and her assistant.

And now, onto your questions…

How messy is home birth? In other words, how many plastic sheets should I buy?

When people hear you're having a home birth, this will be the first concern they have—isn't it going to be so, well, *gross?* I'll confess, before I had a home birth, I pictured *Texas Chainsaw Massacre* with bloody walls and chunky flesh droppings on the carpet. Turns out, it's not that bad. My midwife told me to buy 2 to 3 plastic sheets, so naturally, I bought 6, assuming that I'd drape the whole house in plastic like a scene from some biological contagion movie. But surprisingly, the mess gets pretty well contained.

When you start laboring, you'll probably experience some bleeding—not a problem, just throw on a maxi pad. If your water breaks and it's a gusher, you'll need to do some clean-up, but that could happen even if you were having a hospital birth. During the birth itself, fluids will release. If you're in a tub, it's contained. If you're on the bed, it's contained. And if you're anywhere else, your midwife and assistant will be shoving chux pads underneath your feet to make sure it doesn't get on the carpet. In fact, I think my house was cleaner *after* the birth than it was before.

So don't fret about the mess. You won't even notice it.

If I have a water birth, am I going to be bathing in blood, guts, and gore?

Stop envisioning a scene from *Jaws*. Sure, there will be fluids, maybe even a little blood, but it'll disperse pretty quickly. All the water birthers I spoke to said they didn't even remember a mess.

What should I wear while I'm laboring?

Whatever you want! That's the great part about a home birth. You don't have to trade your comfy clothes for a stiff hospital gown. You can wear your favorite pajamas, a robe, or nothing at all. That's right. You can walk around naked, because it's *your* house. And once you're in the moment, you won't feel bashful at all.

How big should the placenta bowl be?

I had no idea what a placenta looked like or how big it was, so I fretted for months about buying the placenta bowl. The last thing I wanted was some bloody uteral mass slithering out of a too-small bowl and ending up on the carpet. The average placenta is about an inch thick and 9 inches long and weighs about 1 pound. So there you go. A large tupperware or sturdy plastic bowl will work just fine. Happy shopping.

What am I supposed to do with the placenta?

Some midwives might dispose of the placenta for you. Most will just wrap the placenta in plastic and stick it in the freezer. Then you can decide what to do with it—bury it, eat it, encapsulate it for later consumption, or just leave it in the freezer. Technically, you're not supposed to throw it in the garbage. If you're worried, call a biomedical waste management company to handle the disposal.

What the heck is the cookie sheet for?

Your midwife may or may not request this. But some midwives line the cookie sheet with a chux pad and use it as an instrument tray.

And the mirror?

So you can make yourself look fabulous before birthing your baby! Just kidding. If you're interested, you can use the mirror to watch your baby descend from the birth canal.

Um…. olive oil?

If there's one thing you should know about home birth, it's to expect the unexpected. At some point while trying to push out my baby, I realized my midwife was pouring copious amounts of olive oil around my vagina to loosen the perineum and enable my son to slide out more easily. I didn't see that one coming, but it worked, so I won't complain.

I'd like to bank my baby's cord blood. Is this possible with a home birth?

Yes, so long as your midwife feels comfortable collecting the cord blood specimen. If you enroll with one of the big cord banking companies, they'll provide you with a kit and instructions for your midwife on how to collect the cord blood. Check with the company for more details on this process.

Lining Up Your Care Team

Your home birth team includes more than you, your husband, and your midwife. You also need an extensive network of back-up doctors and caregivers. It's a good idea to make contact with these folks well before childbirth to let them know about your plans and to address any issues that might come up.

Midwife's Assistant

Your midwife should have an assistant she brings to the birth. The assistant helps set up the room and acts as a second set of hands. You should try to meet her at some point during the pregnancy so you're not shocked by the stranger in your living room.

Obstetrician

Even in a home birth, you need a back-up obstetrician in case something goes wrong or you decide to pack it in and go to a hospital. In a true emergency during labor, you're going to head to the nearest emergency room and see whomever's on call.

Sometimes, an issue emerges before labor, such as a breech presentation or a baby that's gone past its due date. One home birth mom got into a car accident when she was 38 weeks pregnant and was fortunate to have her back-up doctor lined up. In these unexpected circumstances, you'll need to work with an ob/gyn to assess your options. Your midwife probably has an ob/gyn with whom she works. Set up at least one meeting with the ob/gyn in your last trimester.

Interestingly, meeting with the back-up ob/gyn reassured me. He performed an ultrasound, confirming that the baby was in a good head-down position, and he told me that he'd probably never see me again. I left feeling encouraged and ready to birth at home.

Back-Up Midwife

Every home birther dreads the thought of her midwife being sick or away on vacation when she goes into labor. But your midwife should have another midwife who backs her up under these circumstances. Meet with the back-up midwife in advance just in case she arrives for your birth.

Pediatrician

Although your midwife will do a physical examination of the baby immediately after delivery, you'll need to have a pediatrician see the baby within 24 hours of the birth. Find a pediatrician in advance and meet with him or her to share your plans for a home birth. Ask how flexible his or her office will be in scheduling a last-minute appointment. I find that pediatricians are usually pretty flexible, and if you let them know about your need to see them within 24 hours of the home birth, they'll make themselves available.

Mohel or Ob/Gyn for Circumcision

Giving birth in a hospital makes circumcision easy. The ob/gyn takes the baby off for a quick snip, and you don't have to think about it. But in a home birth, this isn't an option, so if you want your boy circumcised, you need to make arrangements ahead of time. Ob/gyns can perform the procedure, but they don't really have experience in out-of-hospital locations. A better option is to use a mohel, who performs the traditional Jewish circumcision rite.

In reform Judaism, certified mohels are required to be medical professionals, such as ob/gyns, urologists, and certified nurse-midwives, with special training and experience in circumcisions. They routinely perform non-religious circumcisions. The upside to an out-of-hospital circumcision is that mohels go to great lengths to avoid causing discomfort. Many of them do not use artificial restraints, and they often apply local anesthetics to dull the baby's pain. To find a reform mohel, call your local temple for recommendations or go to www.beritmila.org.

Your Birth Plan

Women attempting natural births in a hospital often draft birth plans to formulate their decisions ahead of time so they can clearly articulate them to the hospital staff. These plans are like a childbirth wish list. They allow you to document your preferences, which could include the desire to avoid Pitocin, to move and use different positions during labor, to allow only intermittent fetal monitoring, to have other children present during the birth, and to decline eye ointment for the newborn.

At first, it seems unnecessary to draft a birth plan for a home birth. You're not going to need to fend off an epidural or argue with a nurse over whether you need Pitocin to speed your contractions. These interventions simply won't be available to you. What's more, midwives tend to be very deferential to your preferences. They view themselves as a partner in your birth, not a dictator.

Still, it's a good idea to have a birth plan. Why? Two reasons. One: Even at home, you have to make decisions about who you want in the room, how you want to birth, and what treatments you want for your newborn. Two: In the event you need to transfer to a hospital, you don't want to lose sight of your desire for a natural birth. Having that birth plan handy will help you—and more importantly, your partner— advocate for your preferences.

You can also include instructions for after the birth. In our case, my husband and I had lots of out-of-town relatives flying in, and we were concerned about balancing their desires to maximize time with the baby versus our desire for some occasional privacy. We also didn't want our relatives edging us out of the parenting process. We decided to define clearly what we expected from our post-birth support team.

You should put together the birth plan with your husband in consultation with your midwife. Then be sure to share it with your midwife, doula, and anyone else who might attend the birth.

Below are some questions you may want to ask yourself as you put together your birth plan.

Who should attend my birth?

This totally depends on you. Some mothers want a lot of friends and family around. Others want just their partners and the midwife. At least one midwife requires first-time moms, who are most likely to end up with a hospital transfer, to have no attendees other than the husband and the doula.

Either way, think carefully about who attends. You want people who are supportive of home birth—you don't need any snide comments or panicked outbursts while you're laboring away. You want people who can assist in a meaningful way. And you definitely don't want anyone whose fear might contaminate the birth process.

One home birth mom put it best: "If you don't want someone at the birth, make sure they're not there." It seems simple enough, but feelings can get hurt pretty quickly when you turn someone down. For some reason, people feel entitled to be at your home birth because it's just your house for Pete's sake. It's not like a hospital where they have all sorts of rules about who can visit and be in the room while you birth.

Don't feel obligated to invite someone, and don't be afraid to change your mind. In my first trimester, high off pregnancy hormones and excited about home birth, I invited everyone to witness it. But as the months wore on, I suddenly felt less comfortable with a roomful of spectators and had to uninvite people. It was tough, but it had to be done.

If you have a lot of people, you should consider giving them jobs so they're not just staring at you the whole time. One person can be the videographer. One person can take photos. Another can be in charge of food. These roles actively engage friends and family in your birth experience and let you and your husband focus on the labor.

Your birth plan can include the names of people you want at the birth and their jobs. You should share the plan with them in advance.

Should I have my other children present at the birth?

Again, a personal call. It depends on the age of your children (older children may handle it better) and whether or not they want to be there, if they're old enough to voice an opinion. If a child says he doesn't want to be present, don't force it. But most mothers I spoke to were thrilled to have their other children present, and the kids enjoyed the experience.

Still, it's a good idea to prepare your children for labor and childbirth since it's not something they'll see every day. Here are tips from other moms about getting their children ready for a baby sister/brother born at home:

- Read books about home birth. There are some great children's picture books about home birth that can help start the discussion. *Mama, Talk About When Max Was Born* by Toni Olson and *We're Having a Homebirth!!* by Kelly Mochel are two of the most popular ones. As you read the books, let your child ask questions.

- Sign your child up for a childbirth preparation class just for kids, if there's one in your area.

- Show your child pictures of his birth, if you have them, to open up a dialogue about what he might see.

- Talk about the pain. For a child, seeing her mother in pain could be the most distressing part of the experience, so don't overlook this discussion. One mother told her son that the baby was going to squeeze Mommy's body; it would hurt for a little while, but then the squeezing would stop. They practiced squeezing each other's arms to simulate the pressure and release that occurs in labor.

- Make some noise. You can vocalize the sounds you might utter in labor—groans, grunts, and sighs—so your child isn't surprised by them.

- Have a dry run. Show your child the birthing pool, and walk her through what might happen once you're in labor. Let her know she may see blood, but it doesn't mean you're hurt.

Also, plan to have someone at the birth (other than your partner) to watch your child. That way, you'll only have to worry about the task at hand. Your child should know and trust this person. If your child starts to become upset, the person can take him to another room. You'll also need this person around in case you need to go to the hospital.

Birth is a beautiful family experience, but every child is different, and some may handle it better than others. So be mindful of your child's preferences, not just yours.

What happens if I transfer to a hospital?

Have copies of your birth plan handy in case you need to transfer to a hospital. Depending on the circumstances, you still may want to pursue a natural birth. And don't think just because you're going to the hospital, you're doomed to a c-section. You don't lose all control. You don't check your rights at the door.

Your birth plan can include preferences about Pitocin administration, epidurals, fetal heart monitoring, and episiotomies. And you should make clear to the hospital staff that you want to be able to approve all interventions, from inserting an IV line to upping the Pitocin dose. At the very least, you'd like a few minutes to talk about it with your partner before the hospital staff forges ahead.

Of course, be realistic and flexible. If you're going to the hospital, it's because you need or want some additional support, so don't expect the hospital staff to replicate a home birth environment. That's not what they do. And that's not what you need at the moment.

What treatments should I allow for my newborn?

All states require or strongly recommend two treatments immediately after birth: eye prophylaxis and a Vitamin K injection.

The eye prophylaxis—an antibiotic ointment or drops applied to your newborn's eyes usually within a few hours of birth—guards the baby against blindness in case you're infected with gonorrhea.

The Vitamin K injection prevents a rare but serious bleeding problem called hemorrhagic disease of the newborn (HDN). Babies are born with low levels of Vitamin K, an essential component of blood clotting.

If your state mandates eye prophylaxis and Vitamin K, your midwife will be required to administer them. Almost all states, however, have a religious exemption, and 19 states permit a philosophical exemption. If you're opposed to these treatments, your midwife can provide you with the procedures to request an exemption.

Your midwife can give you alternatives to these treatments, such as oral Vitamin K or supplementing your own diet with Vitamin K-rich foods. She also can arrange for a gonorrhea test before the birth to make sure you're not infected.

7

OH BOY, HERE WE GO…

The birth kit is ready. You've practiced your relaxation breathing. The midwife is on speed dial. And then it hits. The first contraction.

It's show time.

Since every labor is different, it's impossible to map out what yours will look like. But what follows is a general guide to birthing at home— when to call the midwife, when to break out the birth ball, and when to breathe a sigh of relief as you cradle your new baby.

The Play By Play

Labor begins.

You'll want to give your midwife a heads up that you've started laboring so she can rearrange appointments and plan her schedule. But use some common sense. If it's 2 o'clock in the morning, don't call and wake her whole family because you've had a single contraction, unless you have a history of rapid progression. On the other hand, if your water breaks, call your midwife no matter what the time.

And if you think something's wrong (beyond the fact that your cervix is stretching to inhuman proportions), don't be afraid to pick up the phone. Midwives would rather hear from you and assess the situation than overlook a critical component of your care.

At the start of labor, call your doula if you have one. She can help evaluate your needs and get the room ready for a birth.

Once you're in labor, start setting up the room. Take the two sets of sheets out of your birth kit. Place the nicer sheets on the bed. Cover them with a plastic shower curtain or plastic tablecloth (or, if you're as neurotic as I am, two plastic coverings). On top of the plastic, place the old junky sheets. After the birth, you'll toss the junky sheets and plastic and have a fresh set of sheets for you to sleep on.

Get out your comfort aids and start using them, if necessary.

If you're planning a water birth, set up the birth tub if you haven't done so already. You may not need to start filling it yet, but get everything ready to go. Your husband or doula should assist with the set-up.

First, set up the tub itself. Inflating it should only take 15 minutes or so. Then, place the disposable liner inside. Step into the tub with your shoes off and scoot your feet around until the liner is evenly distributed around the tub. Remember to set up the tub in the location you're going to use it, and make sure that location is close enough to a faucet to permit filling.

To fill the tub, hook up the hose with the universal sink connector to the faucet and place the other end in the tub. Turn on the water, checking the temperature periodically. It should be about 100°F. Fill the tub until your abdomen is completely covered. You might want to leave a little extra room at the top so you can pour in more hot water as time allows.

Try to eat and drink as much as you can. And it sounds incredible, but if you're able to, get some sleep. I still can't believe it, but I was actually able to catch some rest between contractions. Take advantage of it.

As you labor, try different positions. Get in and out of the bath. Watch television. Do whatever you need to feel comfortable. The great part about home birth is that you can move around, eat, drink, sleep, and test out different positions as much as you want.

That said, don't be wedded to a particular game plan. I thought I'd be swaying side to side on the birth ball, slow dancing with my husband, and walking around the house. In reality, my most comfortable position was in bed on my back, which I easily could've done in a hospital. The point is—I had a choice.

Feel free to call your midwife and give her updates or have someone else do it for you. Be specific. Let her know how long and how far apart your contractions are. Definitely call if the pressure changes, your water breaks, something just doesn't feel right, or if you have questions.

The midwife arrives.

At some point, the midwife will arrive. She'll check your vital signs. She'll listen to the baby's heartbeat with a fetal Doppler and give you a vaginal exam to see how far along you are. If you're just a few centimeters and don't seem to be progressing quickly, she'll probably go home. She'll likely give you instructions to call if your water breaks or if the pressure changes.

If you're close to giving birth, the midwife will stay. She'll call her assistant, and then it's go time.

It's time!

The midwife and her assistant will set up. They'll unpack your birth kit and lay out all the instruments. They'll test and arrange the midwife's medical supplies, which include oxygen, Pitocin, sutures, and resuscitation equipment. Everything will be organized so the midwife has quick and easy access to anything she might need. You probably won't even know this is going on.

When you're ready, you'll start pushing. Your midwife may have you try different positions, such as squatting beside the bed with your partner supporting you. Or you may lie on your side with your legs pulled back. The midwife might position the mirror so you can witness the baby coming down the birth canal, or she might show you how to reach down and catch your baby.

To reduce the risk of tearing, your midwife might tell you to stop pushing at certain points so she can loosen the perineum muscles with lubrication or olive oil. Follow her lead.

And then…your baby is here!

Welcome your new child.

Don't be surprised if the baby doesn't cry. My son was quiet for a few minutes, very calm and relaxed, just taking things in. That's pretty common in a home birth. Your midwife will place the baby on your chest, and you can say hello for the first time.

Your midwife may or may not cut the cord right away. If you have a preference, you can express this to your midwife in advance. But don't make the same mistake I did. I was so excited to be holding our new baby and wanted my husband to share in the joy that I started handing off the little guy before the cord was cut. Fortunately, my midwife stopped me with a "Wait! He's still attached!"

A few minutes after the birth, the placenta will emerge. Your midwife will place the placenta in the bowl (yay! it fits!) and take it into better light to examine it. She'll check to make sure it's intact because pieces left behind could prevent the uterus from contracting back to position, which will cause bleeding. She'll also look for any anomalies. If everything looks good, she'll probably wrap it up and stick it in your freezer.

Your midwife will perform another vaginal exam and make sure your uterus is contracting normally back into shape. If you had some perineal tearing, your midwife will suture you.

Check the baby.

Your midwife will perform a quick physical examination of the baby. She'll weigh and measure him. And she'll do an Apgar test, which is commonly used in the hospital to assess whether the baby needs immediate medical attention. The Apgar score, a number from 0 to 10, is based on appearance, pulse rate, reflexes, muscle tone, and breathing. Scores of 7 to 10 are generally considered normal.

Your midwife also will place an antibiotic ointment on your baby's eyes and administer a Vitamin K injection, if you have not requested an exemption.

Break out the breast.

You'll want to start breastfeeding right away, and your midwife will encourage it. If you're new to breastfeeding, she'll give you some instruction, and she probably won't leave until the baby is feeding and you're comfortable.

Wrap up loose ends.

Before the midwife and her assistant leave, they'll straighten up. Anything contaminated with fluids will get bagged and dumped. They'll empty the birthing tub by first clearing out any debris and then reversing the hose to drain into your bathtub or toilet.

Afterwards, your midwife will fill out some paperwork, including a record of the birth with all relevant information about your health and the baby's health. You'll need this paperwork when you apply for a birth certificate.

You can expect your midwife to stay with you 2 to 3 hours post-partum. Before leaving, your midwife will check your family one last time. Then, she'll wish you well and give you time to rest and bond with your new baby.

But What If...

I've laid out the ideal home birth, which is what happens most of the time. But sometimes, things don't go as planned.

Maybe your labor stalls out, and you've been dilated at 4 centimeters for seven hours. Maybe you've been pushing for three hours with no progress. Or, maybe you're having a very long, or particularly uncomfortable, labor, and you've had it. You want to go to the hospital. You want that epidural. You, your partner, and your midwife will have a discussion about next steps. You might be able to change positions and get things going again. Maybe you just need some rehydrating fluids. But you should prepare yourself for the fact that you might need to go to the hospital.

Overwhelmingly, first-time moms are most likely to transfer. One study showed that transfer rates were about 40% for first-time mothers compared to about 10% for those who'd previously had children. The most common reason for going to the hospital was failure to progress.

If you decide to go to the hospital for a non-emergency reason (such as stalling out or becoming exhausted), your midwife should accompany you. She will present the hospital staff with your prenatal records and update them on the progress of your labor. But remember that home-birth midwives are not permitted to practice medicine, and most have no hospital privileges. They cannot intervene on your behalf. They cannot give orders to or even communicate with the hospital staff regarding your condition. In the hospital, your midwife effectively becomes a doula.

Some midwives will stay until the baby is born. Depending on the circumstances, other midwives might leave you in the good care of the hospital staff if there are no emergent issues. If your midwife leaves, she'll undoubtedly call to see how you are, and it's a good idea to let your midwife know the outcome of your experience. She'll want to know about your health and the baby's health, and she can continue to treat you post-birth.

Some circumstances may warrant a transfer to the hospital with more urgency. These situations tend to involve less discussion. Under the following situations while you're in labor, your midwife may advise you to go to the hospital:

- labor before 37 weeks
- signs of preeclampsia
- persistent fever over 100.4 degrees
- breech presentation
- evidence of the baby's distress as indicated by a weak fetal heart rate
- abnormal amount of bleeding before delivery
- moderate or thick meconium (baby's first bowel movement)
- suspected placental abruption
- suspected uterine rupture
- seizure
- exhaustion
- unexplained pain
- prolapsed cord

There are times you might make it through the labor just fine, but something goes awry in the aftermath. Here are some reasons you might need to go to the hospital after you've given birth:

- significant postpartum hemorrhage unresponsive to treatment
- retained placenta (there's been more than an hour of active bleeding, and the midwife is unable to remove the placenta manually)
- perineal tear beyond the midwife's ability to repair
- unexplained significant pain
- seizure
- anaphylaxis

With some of these circumstances, such as exhaustion or fever, you can probably have someone drive you to the nearest hospital. (Do I have to tell you not to drive yourself? Seems obvious, but okay: Don't drive yourself). Other situations, such as a prolapsed cord, severe hemorrhaging, or maternal seizure, will demand a 911 call to get you to the emergency room as fast as possible. Your midwife will decide what's best.

It may be the case that you're okay, but your newborn needs immediate medical attention. Generally, your midwife will recommend a trip to the hospital if any of the following occur in your baby:

- seizure
- respiratory distress
- Apgar score of less than 7 at five minutes of age and not improving
- obvious congenital abnormalities
- birth injury requiring medical attention
- poor color or unstable temperature

Your midwife will continue to treat you and the baby until help arrives or until you arrive at the hospital. She's trained for emergencies, and she knows what to do. If you're hemorrhaging, she might start an IV line or administer Pitocin to get the uterus contracting. She can suture a perineal tear. She'll attempt to remove a placenta manually if it doesn't come out on its own. She's armed with resuscitation equipment and oxygen for you and the baby.

Many times, you won't even know that an emergency is underway. One doula reported that at her first home birth, the mother started hemorrhaging after a particularly difficult posterior delivery. The midwife and assistant immediately started an IV line, which stabilized the mother. "At the time, I had no idea a true life-threatening emergency was happening. There was no screaming, no yelling. Not until later did I realize that it was so dangerous," she said.

In other words, you'll receive good care at home, en route to the hospital, or while waiting for paramedics to arrive. In emergency situations, you should expect your midwife to stay at the hospital until you and your baby are safe.

It's understandable if you don't want to go to the hospital. After all, that's what you've been trying to avoid for nine months. But if your midwife says you need a hospital, get in the car. At that point, your midwife knows that your best chance of survival and recovery is not at home. Be thankful we live in a modern, civilized society with access to state-of-the-art medical facilities that will save your life.

And remember, there's nothing wrong with going to the hospital.

"Just because you go to the hospital doesn't mean it was a failed home birth. It just means that it was a non-emergency transfer. And if it's an emergency, it's an emergency," said one home birther, whose first two planned home births ended in hospital transfers due to exhaustion and stalled dilation. Her third child was born at home, proof that prior experiences shouldn't deter you from attempting another home birth under the right circumstances.

Keep positive, even if it's not the birth you pictured.

One mother planning a home birth had to reorient her thinking when her water broke five-and-a-half weeks early. Fortunately, her sister (another home birther) led the mantra: "Same birth, different location, same birth, different location." The mom ended up delivering in the hospital vaginally, all natural, 26 hours after her membranes ruptured.

Her baby was fine, and they all went home the next day.

8

SO NOW WHAT?

For me, the most terrifying part of home birth was when my midwife packed up and left. I was a first-time mother, and the thought of being left alone with this squirming, helpless creature was overwhelming. Home birthers, unlike our hospital-birthing counterparts, don't have a team of nurses standing by to help out, and we don't have the option of sending our newborns to the nursery for a few hours so we can get some sleep. Once that baby comes out, it's nonstop action.

For that reason, it's a good idea to have some postnatal support in addition to your partner—a post-partum doula, your mother-in-law, a friend, basically whoever's willing to pitch in—because there's still a lot to do. Some midwives even require that you have assistance lined up, knowing the pressures are so intense.

Here's your guide for surviving the first few weeks after a home birth.

First Few Hours

Take it easy. Take it easy. Take it easy.

You'll be pumped up on adrenaline and might feel as if you could lift a train off its track. But your body will object if you try.

First things first, especially if you've had a long labor, eat something. You'll be shocked how hungry you are. Immediately after I gave birth, my mother plunked down an overcooked microwave lasagna. It was the most amazing thing I'd ever eaten. I devoured the whole thing within minutes.

Second, don't rush to get up. Your body has been through a lot. You may have lost a lot of blood, and if you get up too fast, you'll feel woozy and could pass out.

I lost a fair amount of blood during labor, and the second I sat up, my head started swimming. The midwife put me in adult diapers and told me to stay horizontal until I regained my equilibrium. I was mortified at the thought of soiling myself, so I dismissed her advice and tried to make it to the bathroom on my own. Immediately, I felt light-headed and the room began to blacken. My mother, ever the voice of calm, started yelling, "Call 911!" Fortunately, I had enough wits to put my head between my legs and get some blood flow back to my brain. I crawled back to the bed and didn't leave for a while.

Which brings me to my next point: listen to your midwife.

If she tells you to piss in a diaper, do it. Your health and the baby's health are her top priority, and she's been through enough of these births to know what's best.

If over the next few hours, you think something's wrong (for example, if you start bleeding heavily) or you just don't feel right, call your midwife right away.

First Few Days

Take the baby to the pediatrician for a physical exam within 24 hours of the birth. You may also need your pediatrician to fill out some paperwork verifying that he or she saw the baby and could attest to its health. This report is required in some states and at least will come in handy when requesting a birth certificate.

Your midwife will come by for a follow-up visit within the first 72 hours. She'll do another vaginal exam and check your vitals. Be sure to share with her any concerns or questions you might have.

You should flush your perineum with tea tree oil if your midwife has instructed you to do so.

Your body will continue to discharge lochia—a mix of blood and placental debris—for up to six weeks after the birth. You may even pass some pretty gnarly blood clots. This isn't cause for concern. Just wear a maxi pad until the bleeding subsides.

Most importantly, bond with your baby. Breastfeed. And try to get rest.

Over the Next Few Weeks

The activity picks up over the next few weeks. If you'd had a hospital birth, your baby would have received several tests before leaving. These tests are required in almost every state, but you can typically request an exemption. You'll have to check with your midwife for your state's specific exemption requirements and procedures. To see the laws in your state, visit the National Newborn Screening and Genetics Resource Center's Web site. They have a great matrix showing all of the testing requirements by state. I've also included some information at the end of the book.

Newborn Screening

This pinprick blood test screens for dozens of genetic disorders, including phenylketonuria (PKU), a rare condition in which a baby is born without the ability to properly break down an amino acid called phenylalanine. If left untreated, PKU can lead to brain damage. All 50 states require the newborn blood screen. Your midwife or pediatrician will perform the screen unless you request an exemption.

Newborn Hearing Screen

Thirty-six states and the District of Columbia require a non-invasive hearing screen. About 3 in 1,000 newborns are born with hearing loss. If undetected, hearing loss can lead to speech and developmental delays. The screen is typically performed in the hospital, but your pediatrician can recommend an audiologist to conduct the test. To see the laws in your state, visit the National Conference of State Legislatures at www.ncls.org or check out the table at the end of the book.

Hepatitis B Vaccine

Babies usually receive the first dose of the Hepatitis B vaccine in the hospital. It's not a big deal to miss out on this one. Your pediatrician can administer the first dose during your baby's first round of immunizations.

Circumcision

If you've decided to have your boy circumcised, you should contact the doctor or mohel to perform the procedure.

Follow-Up Visits

You'll have your final visit with the midwife about 6 weeks after the birth. She'll give you another exam to make sure everything's okay. She'll ask you how breastfeeding is going. And she'll want to see pictures of that cute little baby if you didn't bring the real thing along.

If applicable, make sure to talk to your midwife about birth control before returning to sexual activity. She can prescribe you a birth control option that won't interfere with breastfeeding or refer you to a health professional who can do the same.

And who knows? You may decide to keep seeing your midwife for routine well-woman care. It's a great way to stay in touch and a refreshing change from the cold, sterile stirrups of your ob/gyn's office.

78

9

THE INCONVENIENCE OF A CONVENIENT BIRTH

Having a home birth is really convenient. There's no need to pack a bag. There's no frantic rush to the hospital. You can walk around in your pajamas (or nothing at all) if you want. But the aftermath of home birth is extremely inconvenient.

Turns out, hospitals take care of a lot more than just delivering babies. They make sure you get a birth certificate and a Social Security number for your baby. They bill the insurance company and deal with the paperwork. You'll need to do all of these things on your own.

Your midwife will provide guidance, but there's still a lot of legwork. Here are a few ways to start.

What documentation will I need?

Almost all states require proof that an out-of-hospital birth occurred under the supervision of a licensed health professional. Your midwife should provide you with a record of the birth. This record will certify that you were pregnant and delivered a live baby. It may also include details of the birth, such as whether there were any complications.

Make sure your midwife provides her license number on the form and signs it.

Your pediatrician may also need to fill out a form verifying that he or she saw the baby and found the baby to be in good health.

Because you didn't go to a hospital, this record is all you have. You'll need it to get a birth certificate and Social Security number for your baby. So keep it in a safe place.

How do I get a birth certificate?

Your midwife should have all of the information on how to get a birth certificate in your state. If you have additional questions, contact your local registrar-recorder or your state's vital records department.

In some states, midwives are required to file the paperwork on your behalf. If it's left in your hands, be sure not to dilly dally. The birth certificate is a critical document enabling you to get a Social Security number and insurance coverage for your infant.

Though it depends on your state, you generally need to present the following evidence:

- application for a birth certificate
- proof of your identity and your husband's identity, usually with your driver's licenses
- the midwife's report from the home birth
- the pediatrician's verification of a live birth
- proof of residency, such as a recent utility bill
- the baby

Verify the requirements with your midwife and make sure you have everything you need before going down to your local registrar's office.

Once you've gone through the process, be sure to get a *certified* copy of the birth certificate. You'll need it for everything else.

How do I get a Social Security number?

First, you'll need your baby's birth certificate. Then, you'll need to take the following items to your local Social Security office (despite what the application says, I strongly recommend against mailing the information—I did this and the Social Security Administration lost my passport):

- application for a Social Security number (Form SS-5)
- a certified copy of your baby's birth certificate
- the midwife's report from the home birth
- your U.S. passport or immigration documents

Before you schlep yourself down to the Social Security office, which is a miserable experience, double-check and then triple-check that you have all the documents. You don't want to spend four hours waiting in the Social Security office only to be turned away for missing one document.

Once you've turned everything in, it can take 6 to 8 weeks to receive your baby's Social Security card in the mail. You can find more information at www.ssa.gov.

Can I claim my baby on my taxes if we don't yet have a Social Security number?

Even if your baby is born at the end of the year, you should have time to get a birth certificate and Social Security number before April 15, although you'll need to hustle. We didn't have our son's Social Security number by tax time (see previous answer about Social Security Administration losing my passport), so we left that section blank. The IRS followed up, and by that time, we had a Social Security number to put on the tax form. Worst case scenario is that you file an amended tax return once you have all the information. Contact a tax professional for details.

Will my insurance cover a home birth?

The short answer is…it depends.

The major insurance carriers do not cover home birth unless your state requires them to pay for it (check the table at the end of the book to see if your state requires it). But many insurance companies cover gynecological and well-woman care provided by midwives, particularly certified nurse-midwives.

At the end of the pregnancy and birth, your midwife will hand you a superbill that covers everything—the prenatal visits, the actual birth, and the postnatal visits. It's one fixed fee. Most ob/gyns do the same thing. The home birth itself is not a line item, and it cannot be broken out.

You can submit this bill to your insurance company and see if they'll pay it. Again, you'll have a much better chance if you've used a licensed midwife and, even better, a certified nurse-midwife. If your midwife is out of network, the insurance company will reimburse you for their normal coverage, usually 50% of the usual and customary fee.

You're lucky if your midwife is willing to handle the insurance billing for you. If, like most midwives, she doesn't get involved, you'll need to contact your insurance company to find out how to place a claim.

Any advice on covering the costs of a home birth?

The cruddy part about home birth is that even though it costs way less than a hospital birth, you'll probably end up paying more out of pocket than your hospital-birthing friends. That's because insurance covers hospital births without a second thought. But home births are a no-go. So you'll need to get creative.

First, ask your midwife whether she'll consider a payment plan. She may let you pay off the total tab in a few installments throughout the pregnancy or even after the birth.

Second, consider setting up a flexible spending account (FSA) or health savings account (HSA) through your employer or a local bank. Your tax adviser can give you the details. These accounts allow you to set aside pre-tax earnings for eligible medical expenses.

Generally, midwifery services are a covered expense. If your insurance company covers only part of your midwife's fee, the FSA/HSA may pick up the remainder. If your insurance company refuses to cover any part of the midwife's services, it may be a hard sell to get reimbursed from the FSA/HSA, but it's worth a shot. The standards of eligibility and coverage tend to be lower with these tax deferred accounts.

Additionally, your FSA/HSA may cover other home birth-related costs, including:

- laboratory fees
- prenatal tests
- birth kit ordered from a medical supply provider
- childbirth classes, such as Lamaze and Bradley Method (HypnoBirthing may or may not be eligible)
- breast pumps and lactation supplies

In some cases, your midwife or physician may need to write you a letter of medical necessity to prove you need the items. Submitting a claim to your FSA/HSA isn't a guarantee you'll get reimbursed, but again, there's no harm in asking.

Can my midwife fill out my disability paperwork? How about my maternity leave paperwork?

Yes, a licensed midwife has the authority to sign your disability and maternity leave paperwork. The location of your birth has no bearing on your leave of absence.

10

ADVICE FOR YOUR PARTNER

Originally, I wanted my husband to write this chapter. I was hoping he could speak frankly to home birth dads in a way I never could—you know, man to man. But my husband listened to my pitch, politely nodded his head, and declined. Ah, well. I wasn't surprised.

For one, he's not a great writer. And two, even when we were planning a home birth, my husband was far less engaged than I was.

For good reason.

Even though it was our baby, it was my body, and I wanted (and deserved) a bigger say. After all, my husband wasn't going to be the one battling Pitocin contractions or getting poked and prodded by overzealous nurses in a hospital birth. So he naturally deferred to my preferences.

That said, my husband was always supportive of a home birth. We had both watched *The Business of Being Born*, and together made the decision to have our son at home. This unity was critical. You simply must have a partner who supports a home birth. Forging ahead with a reluctant—or worse, hostile—partner is simply untenable.

Your husband's experience with a home birth will be completely different from yours. You will be completely focused on the task at hand—breathing through each contraction, trying to get comfortable, bringing your baby into the world. Imagine yourself as the diva who needs to sing and look pretty. Meanwhile, your husband is sweating it out behind the scenes to make sure you have a flawless performance. He's ensuring that you stay hydrated, helping you in and out of the tub, rubbing your back, supporting you in various positions. You couldn't do it without him.

Your job is fairly clear—having the baby. But your husband may not understand the critical role he will play in a home birth. Just like you, he'll have a lot of questions.

Here's an attempt to answer them from dads who've been through the process before.

What's my role in a home birth?

You're the birth partner. Unlike the midwife, who is the medical authority monitoring heartbeats and ensuring the safety of your family, your job is to support your wife. This means do whatever you need to do to keep her happy and comfortable, or as my husband would say, it's business as usual. You are her emotional support and her physical support.

When I was laboring, it was helpful to know my husband was there, even if he wasn't doing anything. I just wanted him around, rubbing my legs, watching television, whatever. Honestly, we women don't need much in labor, and when we're busy breathing and focusing on relaxation, we're far less high maintenance than usual. Basically, your role is just to be you.

Okay, seriously, what am I supposed to do?

Most men shine during home births, because unlike in hospital births—in which you might feel intimidated or worse alienated by the hospital staff—the home is your castle. You're in your element. You know how everything works. You know where all the stuff is. This confidence allows you to focus on what you do best: logistics.

Your wife will be in no shape to worry about the practical details. That's where you come in. Here are some things over which you can take charge:

- Set up the birth pool (no power tools required).

- Unpack the birth kit and help get the room ready for a birth.

- Time the contractions. You probably learned in childbirth class how to time the length and frequency of contractions to gauge your wife's progress—break out the stopwatch!

- Offer your wife food and water even if she doesn't ask for it and especially if she's having a long labor. My husband was relentless in shoving coconut water and yogurt in my face. Most of the time I refused, but every once in a while, I'd give in, which was a good thing, because it helped keep my energy levels up.

- Go into coaching mode. In childbirth class, you learned how to assist your wife through labor. You probably learned prompts to refocus her breathing and some relaxation techniques, such as massage. Now's the time to put that hard-earned knowledge to use. It's very likely your wife will get distracted and forget what she has learned. That's why she needs you to set her back on track. Go through the motions just as they taught you in childbirth class.

- Provide physical support. You might be able to assist your wife in certain comforting positions, such as the slow dance (your wife's arms are draped around you as though you're dancing) or the supported squat (hold her torso up as she squats down). When it comes time to push, you can help keep her legs open or bear down with her into a squat.

- Be the brains. Your wife may not be thinking straight. Case in point: When the midwife arrived around my 25th hour of labor, I was at my wit's end. She did a vaginal exam and pronounced me 9 centimeters dilated. "Wow, that's great," I said. "So do you want to go home, and I'll call you when I get closer to pushing?" Clearly, I was a little out of it, assuming that my midwife would leave with a mere centimeter to go. That's why we need you to have a clear head. Your straight thinking will come in especially handy if there's talk of transferring to a hospital or employing an intervention.

- Delegate. Your job is to focus on your wife's needs. If you have other support around, such as a doula or helpful friends and family, put them to work. If your midwife asks for the olive oil, assign someone to be the runner. If you need more hot water for the birthing tub, delegate the responsibility to someone nearby.

Even if your wife doesn't say it, she appreciates everything you're doing. Believe me, we will be overcome by the love we feel for you once it's all over.

My wife keeps yelling at me. I don't think she wants me around.

Don't take anything your wife says too personally when she's in labor. She's under a lot of stress, and she's lost her mind (see previous answer regarding "no brains.") She loves you. She wants you there. Don't start an argument with her.

Our childbirth coach told me to massage my wife to help her relax, but every time I touch her, she snaps at me. What gives?

We can't predict how we're going to feel in labor. Be flexible and respond to your wife's cues. In HypnoBirthing, my husband learned to use light-touch massage as a relaxation technique. But when I was in labor, the light-touch massage made my skin crawl. I wanted brute force. So he had to adapt. No biggie. Don't get discouraged. Just go with it. Sometimes the game plan changes.

My wife just told me she couldn't do it anymore. How do I know if she just needs encouragement or if it's time to go to the hospital?

Oftentimes, women reach a point where they say, "I can't do this anymore." It usually means they're very close to the pushing phase. First, offer encouragement and reassurance. Then, get an expert opinion. Your midwife can assess your wife's progress. If your wife's been stalled out for a while and shows no sign of advancing, you should discuss next steps. But the midwife might tell you she's 8 centimeters dilated and progressing quickly, indicating that your wife's plea for help was just a bit of normal self-doubt. It's important that you don't express the same doubts. Your wife is counting on you to be strong. Stay by her side, give her encouragement, and tell her she's almost there.

I've never seen a birth before. I'm worried I might freak out, or worse, pass out.

The best way to prepare for a birth is to watch one. There are hundreds of home birth videos on YouTube. Or rent *The Business of Being Born* or any other documentary about home birth. And recognize that your child's birth will be infinitely more satisfying than the births of those strangers.

For that reason alone, you probably won't freak out. Your wife and baby are depending on you, and nothing brings out the best in men more than the innate desire to protect and keep safe their family.

That said, there are men who get squeamish or lightheaded or just plain overwhelmed by the situation. You'll need to get a doula for extra support. There's no shame in recognizing your limitations. If you're worried about how you'll react, it's far better to let someone else chip in than to let your wife flounder.

It sounds gross to be in the birthing tub with my wife. Won't it be filled with fluids and blood?

Yes, there might be some fluids. There might be some blood. But trust me, you won't notice it. Because also in that tub are your wife and soon-to-be-born child, and if you had to walk through a sludge of fetid body parts to get to them, you would.

Apparently, during the birth of our son, some fluids splashed onto my husband's leg. Ordinarily, this would have sent him into a fit of dry heaves. But he never even mentioned it until a few weeks ago. Why? Because it mattered so little at the time.

My wife wants me to catch our baby. But I'm not sure I'm really up for the task. What should I tell her?

This is all about your comfort level. Some men want to catch the baby or cut the umbilical cord. Others don't. If you have reservations, let your wife and midwife know in advance. You also can include your preferences in the birth plan. But remember, you might feel differently in the moment. My husband was dead set against cutting the cord until the midwife stuck the clamps in his hand. Then he snipped away.

Is it okay for me to sleep for a few hours while she's in labor?

Sure, if you want to have it thrown in your face for the next five years. Here's the thing: unless you're the kind of guy who can pull back-to-back all-nighters (like my husband), you're going to need some rest, especially during a long labor. But your wife is not going to appreciate you snoozing in the next room while she's grunting and swearing through every contraction and *having your baby* for goodness sake. She wants you there, even if you're not doing anything. Just be there. And if you can't be there for the long haul, hire a doula. You and the doula can switch off so you both get some rest, and your wife can have someone with her at all times.

What if the doula tries to take over my role as the birth partner?

She won't, but if you're concerned, talk to her about it. Doulas are trained to strike the perfect balance between being helpful and not interfering with your role. But before you hire a doula, discuss these issues with her and make sure each of your roles is clear.

How can I support my wife after the birth?

This may be the most critical time. Your wife will be flooded with hormones and may even get the baby blues. You should plan to stay home with her and the baby for at least a week, more if you can swing it. Also, reach out to friends and family for assistance in the first few weeks. While you're supporting your wife and new baby, others can pitch in with the cleaning, cooking, and caring for your other children.

Allow me to put back on my woman's hat for one last point. Some men (my husband included) struggle with their sensitive, emotional side and may feel out of sorts during the birth experience, especially one as free and natural as home birth.

But most women will tell you that there is nothing manlier or sexier than watching their guys in action at a natural home birth. There's nothing wussy or granola about it. Nothing says "man" more than a guy applying Chapstick to his wife's lips, spooning applesauce into her mouth, or catching his own baby.

11

FROM MOTHER TO MOTHER

What home birth book wouldn't be complete without the obligatory, uplifting birth stories?

I spoke to many midwives, doulas, and childbirth educators while researching this book. But my favorite interviews came from the other moms who had birthed at home. Some of them had such incredible stories, I wish I could print them all verbatim. But this book is about practical advice, so I've restrained myself.

When you're having a hospital birth, you'll get plenty of tips from other moms on what to expect. Home birthers rarely have an extended community to which they can turn.

So this is for you, your mother-to-mother advice.

On having support

"My husband was a home birth, so he wasn't afraid. I didn't have to fight with my husband that this was a crazy idea. It's a lot to take on when you think you're doing it on your own. Women don't fight for a home birth when they're not supported."

—Keri, Long Beach, Calif.
Both children born at home. During the birth of her son, she pushed for three hours with no progress. Then, the midwife discovered the baby's hand was blocking the cervix. On the next contraction, the midwife pushed the baby's hand out of the way, and he was delivered moments later. Her daughter was born at home with her son nearby.

On mentally preparing

"I feel like you really need to be in the right mindset, because so much of a home birth is letting go. It's not for everyone. Probably, if you're not of the right mindset, you'll just hit that threshold."

—Janelle, Manhattan Beach, Calif.
First child born in the hospital. Second child born at home.

On the importance of a birth plan

"Home birth moms, oftentimes when they get to the hospital, they feel like they're going to get a c-section. They give up. They all feel like that's where they're going. But it's not out of your hands. I think what a lot of home birth moms don't understand is that it's still your body, and you still have every right to decide every single thing that happens to it."

—Chelsea, Culver City, Calif.
First two births were planned home births resulting in hospital transfers. In the first birth, she labored for six days before going to the hospital. In the second birth, she got stuck in the same place she had with her first birth. Her third child was born at home.

On reactions from others

"I expected lots of people to be down my throat about it being dangerous, but nobody thought that. If they did, they kept it to themselves. I was pleasantly surprised that not anyone challenged me on it."

—Lana, Downey, Calif.
First birth was a natural birth in the hospital. Second child was born at home.

On having your other children at the birth

"I really enjoy having older siblings at the birth of their little brothers and sisters. I think it's wonderful! I have a handout that I give to parents that has to do with preparing older siblings to be present at the delivery. I encourage parents to enroll their older children into childbirth preparation classes that are designed specifically for kids. I also tell them that they need to have another adult with whom the child is familiar be present at the birth in case the older child wishes to not be present at the time of delivery. We don't want to force a child to be present if they do not wish to be. If they change their mind in the moment, they need to have a trusted adult caretaker present, someone other than the mom or her partner."

—Erin Curtiss, LM, Seattle, Wash.

On dealing with unexpected circumstances

"Things can come up unexpectedly in any situation. The important thing is that people feel that they're with a team that can handle unexpected situations. The worst case scenario can happen whether you're at home or in the hospital, and most unexpected situations that occur are handled very well by midwives...We can control how we prepare, and we can control how we respond in the moment. If something goes against the plan or something is unexpected, we have a choice how we respond to that and how we react to the situation."

—Justine, Huntington Beach, Calif., doula and childbirth educator
Both children born at home.

APPENDICES

Birth Kit Checklist

Six weeks before your due date:

Standard birth kit (order online)
- ☐ bulb syringe
- ☐ lubricating jelly
- ☐ cord clamps/tape
- ☐ gloves
- ☐ iodine/hibiclens scrub (antiseptic)
- ☐ sanitary brief
- ☐ various sizes of underpads (chux pads)
- ☐ plastic-backed sheets
- ☐ sanitary pads
- ☐ perineal irrigation bottle
- ☐ gauze
- ☐ alcohol prep pads
- ☐ flexible straws
- ☐ infant tape measure
- ☐ basic infant cotton cap

Additional items:
- ☐ garbage bags
- ☐ freezer bags
- ☐ scissors

- [ ] old towels, wash cloths, and blankets
- [ ] two sets of sheets (you'll throw out one set after the birth)
- [ ] bowl for the placenta
- [ ] cookie sheet
- [ ] 2-3 plastic sheets or shower curtains (disposable plastic-sided tablecloths also work)
- [ ] more lubricant or olive oil
- [ ] more sanitary napkins
- [ ] newborn diapers
- [ ] baby receiving blankets
- [ ] flashlight
- [ ] mirror
- [ ] map to the nearest emergency room
- [ ] contact information for the nearest hospital, back-up obstetrician, and pediatrician
- [ ] birth plan (if you have one)

Three weeks before your due date:

Water birth supplies
- [ ] birthing tub
- [ ] tub liner (buy some extras if you intend to try out the tub before labor)
- [ ] air pump
- [ ] water thermometer
- [ ] small fishing net for light debris removal

Two weeks before your due date:

- [ ] Stocked refrigerator – food for your family and the midwife
- [ ] Gas in the car

Sample Plan for Home Birth

This birth plan will serve as a guide for our labor and delivery. [YOUR NAME AND YOUR PARTNER'S NAME] understand that this plan is based on our best guess of how we might feel at the time, and it is subject to change, even during labor.

About the Birth

We have chosen to have a home birth attended by a midwife. It is our desire to labor in the most natural, comfortable way possible. I will not use any pain medication, and there will be no interventions unless the midwife deems it necessary and appropriate. The midwife is the medical authority during labor, and we will defer to her recommendations at all times.

During Labor

Our overriding priority is to establish the most comfortable, anxiety-free space for our birth and to have ample time as mother and father to bond with our new baby.

We request that there be no mention of pain during labor.

I want to be able to drink and eat if I so choose, and I will have food on hand for that purpose. Others should feel free to help themselves to anything in the kitchen. Please do not allow me to play hostess.

House phones and cell phones will be turned off or to silent during the labor and birth. If you need to make a non-emergency phone call, please step outside.

The following people may be present at the birth:

Name:	*Role:*
[Partner's Name]	Care for me during labor and keep me relaxed and calm.
[Midwife's Name]	Medical authority
[Midwife's Assistant]	Assist the midwife
[Doula]	Provide support to me and my partner
[Other Name]	…
[Other Name]	…

(Other suggested roles:
photographer, videographer, caretaker for other children, etc.)

At all times, those in attendance must be supportive of our decision to have a natural home birth, and they should not at any point question the midwife, make disparaging remarks, or suggest transfer to the hospital. If we ask you to leave the room, please do so without question or argument, and above all, do not be offended.

Emergencies and Hospital Transfers

In the event of an emergency, I will go to [NAME OF CLOSEST HOSPITAL] by private car or ambulance. For non-emergency transfer, I will go to [NAME OF HOSPITAL USED BY BACK-UP OB/GYN].

After the Birth

Immediately after the birth, we want ample time to bond with our new baby.

I wish to attempt breastfeeding as soon as possible.

We will have our baby circumcised eight days after birth with a mohel.

Post-Partum: Up to 2 Weeks After Birth

We are very grateful to have support in the few weeks after birth. During this time, we will take care of each other and the baby, including feedings, changing the diapers and general care, and we will look to our support team for other household tasks, such as the dishes, laundry, cleaning, cooking, running errands, etc. This will be a huge help to us as we bond with our new baby and learn to become parents. Please do not expect us to play host and hostess during this time – we'll have our hands full!

Also, if at any time we request some privacy, please respect our wishes. We may want a day or two with just mother, father and baby. We understand that our support team has traveled a great distance to be here, but we must make our mental health and our baby's well-being our top priority.

Emergency Numbers

Nearest hospital (emergency transfers)
Emergency room phone number
Labor & delivery phone number

Hospital of back-up ob/gyn (non-emergency transfers)
Labor & delivery phone number

Name and phone number of back-up ob/gyn

Name and phone number of pediatrician

Name and phone numbers (work, cell) of husband/birth partner

Name and phone numbers (work, cell) of one emergency contact

Table 1:
Midwife Licensing and Prescription Authority by State

	Licensure Provided			Administer Drugs		Prescribe Drugs	
	CNM	DEM	Eligible Credential	CNM	DEM	CNM	DEM
Alabama	•			•		•	
Alaska	•	•	CPM	•	•	•	
Arizona	•	•	CPM	•	•	•	
Arkansas	•	•	CPM	•		•	
California	•	•	CPM exam	•	•	•	
Colorado	•	•	CPM	•	^	•	
Connecticut	•			•		•	
Delaware	•	•	CPM, CM	•	•	•	
District of Columbia	•			•		•	
Florida	•	•	CPM exam	•	•	•	
Georgia	•			•		•	
Hawaii	•			•		•	
Idaho	•	•	CPM	•	•	•	
Illinois	•			•		•	
Indiana	•			•		•	
Iowa	•			•		•	
Kansas	•			•		•	
Kentucky	•			•		•	
Louisiana	•	•	CPM	•	•	•	
Maine	•	•		•		•	
Maryland	•			•		•	
Massachusetts	•			•		•	
Michigan	•			•		•	
Minnesota	•	•	CPM	•	•	•	
Mississippi	•			•		•	
Missouri	•	•	CPM, CM	•	•	•	

	Licensure Provided			Administer Drugs		Prescribe Drugs	
	CNM	DEM	Eligible Credential	CNM	DEM	CNM	DEM
Montana	•	•	CPM exam	•	•	•	
Nebraska	•			•		•	
Nevada	•			•		•	
New Hampshire	•	•	CPM	•	•	•	
New Jersey	•	•	CPM, CM	•	•	•	
New Mexico	•	•	CPM	•	•	•	
New York	•	•	CM	•	•	•	•
North Carolina	•			•		•	
North Dakota	•			•		•	
Ohio	•			•		•	
Oklahoma	•			•		•	
Oregon	•	•	CPM	•	•	•	
Pennsylvania	•			•		•	
Rhode Island	•		CM	•	•	•	
South Carolina	•	•	CPM	•	•	•	
South Dakota	•			•		•	
Tennessee	•	•	CPM	•		•	
Texas	•	•	CPM	•		•	
Utah	•	•	CPM	•		•	
Vermont	•	•	CPM	•	•	•	
Virginia	•	•	CPM	•		•	
Washington	•	•	CPM exam	•	•	•	
West Virginia	•			•		•	
Wisconsin	•	•	CPM	•	•	•	
Wyoming	•	•		•		•	

Source: *The Big Push for Midwives, various state statutes*

^ Direct-entry midwives can carry oxygen only

Table 2:
Midwifery Insurance Coverage Requirements by State

	Medicaid Reimbursement Required		Private Insurance Coverage Required*	
	CNM	DEM	CNM	DEM
Alabama	•	•	•	
Alaska	•		•	
Arizona	•		•	
Arkansas	•	•	•	
California	•	•	•	
Colorado	•		•	
Connecticut	•		•	
Delaware	•	•	•	^
District of Columbia	•		•	
Florida	•	•	•	
Georgia	•		•	
Hawaii	•		•	
Idaho	•	•	•	
Illinois	•		•	
Indiana	•		•	
Iowa	•		•	
Kansas	•		•	
Kentucky	•		•	
Louisiana	•		•	
Maine	•		•	
Maryland	•		•	
Massachusetts	•		•	
Michigan	•		•	
Minnesota	•		•	
Mississippi	•		•	
Missouri	•	•	•	^
Montana	•		•	

	Medicaid Reimbursement Required		Private Insurance Coverage Required*	
	CNM	DEM	CNM	DEM
Nebraska	•		•	
Nevada	•		•	
New Hampshire	•	•	•	•
New Jersey	•	•	•	^
New Mexico	•	•	•	•
New York	•	•	•	•
North Carolina	•		•	
North Dakota	•		•	
Ohio	•		•	
Oklahoma	•		•	
Oregon	•	•	•	
Pennsylvania	•		•	
Rhode Island	•	•	•	^
South Carolina	•	•	•	
South Dakota	•		•	
Tennessee	•		•	
Texas	•		•	
Utah	•		•	
Vermont	•	•	•	•
Virginia	•		•	
Washington	•	•	•	
West Virginia	•		•	
Wisconsin	•		•	
Wyoming	•		•	

Source: *The Big Push for Midwives, American College of Nurse-Midwives*

* Insurance coverage guaranteed for midwifery services. Does not necessarily mean the insurance company will cover home birth.
^ Certified midwives only.

Table 3:
Newborn Test Requirements and Exemptions by State

	Testing Required				Allowable Exemptions	
	Vit. K	Eye Drops	Hearing Screen	Genetic Screen	Religious	Other
Alabama	•	•	•	•	•	
Alaska	•	•	•	•	•	
Arizona	•	•		•	•	•
Arkansas	•	•	•	•	•	•
California	•	•		•	•	•
Colorado	•	•		•	•	•
Connecticut	•	•	•	•	•	
Delaware	•	•	•	•	•	
District of Columbia	•	•	•	•	•	
Florida	•	•	•	•	•	
Georgia	•	•		•	•	
Hawaii	•	•	•	•	•	
Idaho	•	•		•	•	•
Illinois	•	•	•	•	•	
Indiana	•	•	•	•	•	
Iowa	•	•	•	•	•	
Kansas	•	•	•	•	•	
Kentucky	•	•		•	•	
Louisiana	•	•		•	•	•
Maine	•	•		•	•	•
Maryland	•	•	•	•	•	
Massachusetts	•	•	•	•	•	
Michigan	•	•	•	•	•	•
Minnesota	•	•	•	•	•	•
Mississippi	•	•	•	•		

	Testing Required				Allowable Exemptions	
	Vit. K	Eye Drops	Hearing Screen	Genetic Screen	Religious	Other
Missouri	•	•	•	•	•	•
Montana	•	•	•	•	•	
Nebraska	•	•		•	•	
Nevada	•	•		•	•	
New Hampshire	•	•		•	•	
New Jersey	•	•	•	•	•	
New Mexico	•	•	•	•	•	•
New York	•	•	•	•	•	
North Carolina	•	•	•	•	•	
North Dakota	•	•		•	•	•
Ohio	•	•	•	•	•	•
Oklahoma	•	•	•	•	•	•
Oregon	•	•		•	•	
Pennsylvania	•	•	•	•	•	•
Rhode Island	•	•	•	•	•	
South Carolina	•	•	•	•	•	
South Dakota	•	•		•	•	
Tennessee	•	•	•	•	•	
Texas	•	•		•	•	•
Utah	•	•	•	•	•	
Vermont	•	•	•	•	•	•
Virginia	•	•	•	•	•	
Washington	•	•		•	•	•
West Virginia	•	•	•	•		
Wisconsin	•	•	•	•	•	•
Wyoming	•	•	•	•	•	

Source: National Newborn Screening and Genetics Resource Center, National Conference of State Legislatures

References

American College of Nurse-Midwives, "Standards for the Practice of Midwifery." Revised and Approved September 24, 2011.

Dedercq, Eugene, Ph.D., and Marian F. MacDorman, Ph.D., Fay Menacker, Dr.Ph., and Naomi Stotland, MD. "Characteristics of Planned and Unplanned Home Births in 19 States." *Obstetrics & Gynecology* 116:1 (2010).

Hollowell, Jennifer and David Puddicombe, Rachel Rowe, Louis Linsell, Pollyanna Hardy, Mary Stewart, Maggie Redshaw, Mary Newburn, Christine McCourt, Jane Sandall, Alison Macfarlane, Louise Silverton, Peter Brocklehurst on behalf of the Birthplace in England Collaborative Group. "The Birthplace national prospective cohort study: perinatal and maternal outcomes by planned place of birth." Birthplace in England research programme. Final report part 4, November 2011.

Janssen, Patricia A. PhD, Lee Saxell MA, Lesley A. Page PhD, Michael C. Klein MD, Robert M. Liston MD, Shoo K. Lee MBBS PhD. "Outcomes of planned home birth with registered midwife versus planned hospital birth with midwife or physician." *Canadian Medical Association Journal.* 2009 September 15; 181 (6-7).

Johnson KC and Daviss BA. "Outcomes of planned home births with certified professional midwives: large prospective study in North America." *BMJ.* 2005 Jun 18; 330 (7505):1416.

MacDorman, Marian F. Ph.D., T.J. Mathews, M.S., and Eugene Declercq, Ph.D. "Home Births in the United States, 1990–2009." NCHS Data Brief, No. 84, January 2012.

Maughan, Karen L., MD, and Steven W. Heim, MD, MSPH, and Sim S. Galazka, MD. "Preventing Postpartum Hemorrhage: Managing the Third Stage of Labor." *American Family Physician* 73: 1 (2006): 1025-1028.

Midwifery Accreditation Council. "Frequently Asked Questions for Aspiring Midwife Students." www.meac.org.

Midwives' Association of Washington State. "Indications for Discussion, Consultation and Transfer of Care in an Out-of-Hospital Midwifery Practice," April 24, 2008.

--. "Planned Out-of-Hospital Birth Transfer Guide," April 24, 2008.

National Conference of State Legislatures. "States with Religious and Philosophical Exemptions from School Immunization Requirements," January 2012.

National Newborn Screening and Genetics Resource Center. "National Newborn Screening Status Report," February 15, 2012.

North American Registry of Midwives. "Report of the 2008-2009 Job Analysis and Test Specifications," January 2010.

Waldenstrom, U. and Schytt, E. "A longitudinal study of women's memory of labour pain: from 2 months to 5 years after the birth." *BJOG: An International Journal of Obstetrics and Gynaecology*, 2008.

Wax, Joseph R., MD, and F. Lee Lucas, PhD, Maryanne Lamont, MLS, Michael G. Pinette, MD, Angelina Cartin, Jacquelyn Blackstone, DO. "Maternal and newborn outcomes in planned home birth vs planned hospital births: a metaanalysis." *American Journal of Obstetrics & Gynecology.* September 2010. 203(3): 243.e1-243.e8.

Resources

Midwives

American College of
Nurse-Midwives
www.midwife.org

North American Registry
of Midwives
www.narm.org

Midwives Association
of North America
www.mana.org

Childbirth Education

HypnoBirthing
www.hypnobirthing.com

The Bradley Method
www.bradleybirth.com

Lamaze International
www.lamaze.org

Doulas

DONA International
www.dona.org

Birth Kit Supplies

Cascade HealthCare Products
www.1cascade.com

In His Hands Birth Supply
www.inhishands.com

Index

A

American College of Nurse-
Midwives, 23, 24, 108, 111
amniocentesis, 12, 28, 34
Apgar score, 69, 72
aromatherapy, 21, 41, 47

B

baths, 41, 46
birth ball, 41, 46
birth certificate, 69, 77, 79, 80, 81
birth coach, 22, 42
birth control, 78
birth kit, 12, 51, 52–54, 65, 66, 67,
83, 87, 99
birth plan, 59–60, 90, 101
birth record, 69, 79, 80
birthing stool, 46
blood screens, 33
breastfeeding, 26, 32, 35, 42, 50,
69, 77, 78, 83, 102
breathing, in labor, 42, 43, 44, 45,
47, 65, 69, 86, 87
breech birth, 8, 30, 58, 71

C

caesarean section, 3, 4, 8, 37, 63,
94
certified midwife (CM), 24
certified nurse-midwives, 22, 59,
82
certified professional midwife, 25
childbirth preparation, 41–45

children, at birth, 62, 95
circumcision, 29, 59, 78, 102
CM. *See* certified midwives
CNM. *See* certified nurse-
midwives
comfort aids, 47, 54, 66
contract, midwife, 35, 36
contractions, 38, 44, 48, 65, 86, 87
cord blood, 57
cord prolapse, 4, 8, 71
costs, 12–13, 35, 46, 50, 54
CPM. *See* certified professional
midwife

D

DEM. *See* direct-entry midwives
demographics, home birthers, 16
diabetes, 8, 12, 33
direct-entry midwives, 23, 24, 106
disability, 83
doula, i, 2, 11, 12, 22, 26, 31, 48,
49, 50, 49–50, 60, 66, 70, 72, 75,
88, 89

E

eating, in labor, 52, 54, 87, 100,
101
emergencies, 4, 10, 23, 29, 30, 31,
43, 58, 72, 73, 95, 102, 103
epidural, 4, 9, 15, 18, 31, 37, 38,
40, 41, 59, 70
episiotomy, 4, 21, 32
exhaustion, 71, 73
eye prophylaxis, 59, 63, 69

F

fetal Doppler, 32, 33, 67
fetal heart monitor, 32, 39, 59
fetoscope, 33
first-time mothers, 35, 60, 70, 75
flexible spending account, 82
FSA. *See* flexible spending account
fundal height, 33

G

glucose tolerance test, 33
Group B streptococcus (GBS), 12, 33

H

health savings account, 82
hemorrhage. *See* postpartum hemorrhage
Hepatitis B vaccine. *See* vaccinations
high blood pressure, 8
hospital transfers, 26, 28, 30, 31, 33, 52, 55, 60, 63, 71, 73, 102
HSA. *See* health savings account
HypnoBirthing, 26, 38, 43, 83, 88, 113

I

insurance, 2, 12, 13, 22, 23, 24, 25, 34, 35, 36, 79, 80, 81, 82, 83, 107, 108
interventions, 4, 18, 21, 22, 32, 33, 39, 44, 49, 59, 63, 88, 101
intravenous line, 21, 31, 32, 72

L

labor pains, 31
laboratory tests, 12, 83
Lamaze, 44, 83, 113
lay midwife, 25
liability waiver, 34, 36
licensed midwife, 25, 28, 82, 83
LM. *See* licensed midwife
lochia, 77

M

malpractice insurance, 34, 36
massage, 47, 87, 88
maternity leave, 83
meconium, 71
membranes, rupture of, 4, 32, 67
mess, 55, 56, 89
midwife
  ability to carry drugs, 24
  caseload, 29
  fee, 12
  interview of, 27–28
  licensure, 22–23
  referrals, 26
  types, 22–26
midwife, back-up, 28, 58
midwife's assistant, 10, 12, 28, 35, 54, 55, 57, 67, 69, 72
Midwives Alliance of North America, 23, 26
mohel, 59, 78, 102

N

NARM. *See* North American Registry of Midwives
neighbors, 11
newborn blood screen, 77

ABOUT THE AUTHOR

Renee Moilanen lives in Redondo Beach, Calif., with her husband and son, who was born at home in 2009. She writes a bimonthly column for the *Daily Breeze* newspaper about parenting and young family life, and her articles have appeared in the *Los Angeles Times*, *Daily Breeze*, *Los Angeles Daily News*, and *Reason* magazine.

Made in the USA
Middletown, DE
30 March 2015